D1566570

The History of Radiology

The History
of Radiology

Adrian M.K. Thomas

Arpan K. Banerjee

Series Advisor

Christopher Gardner-Thorpe

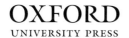

OXFORD

UNIVERSITY PRESS

OXFORD
UNIVERSITY PRESS

Great Clarendon Street, Oxford, OX2 6DP,
United Kingdom

Oxford University Press is a department of the University of Oxford.
It furthers the University's objective of excellence in research, scholarship,
and education by publishing worldwide. Oxford is a registered trade mark of
Oxford University Press in the UK and in certain other countries

© Oxford University Press 2013

The moral rights of the authors have been asserted

First Edition published 2013

Impression: 1

British Library Cataloguing in Publication Data
Data available

ISBN 978–0–19–963997–7

Printed and bound by
CPI Group (UK) Ltd, Croydon, CR0 4YY

To my mother Mary. I still miss you.
To my children, Gareth, Charlotte, and Owen.
I have learnt so much from each of you.

Adrian M.K. Thomas

To my late mother for her selfless devotion to her children.
To my father for his wisdom and continued encouragement.
To my wife, Tina, for her patience and support.
To my daughters, Shonali and Shiuli, for providing
inspiration for the future.

Arpan K. Banerjee

Foreword

This series of Oxford Medical Histories is designed to bring to a wide readership of clinical doctors and others from many backgrounds a short but comprehensive text setting out the essentials of medicine.

History describes the knowledge acquired over time by human beings. It is a form of storytelling, of organizing knowledge, of sorting and giving impetus to information. The study of medical history, just like the history of other human endeavours, enables us to analyse our knowledge of the past in order to plan our journey forward and hence try to limit repetition of our mistakes—a sort of planned process of Natural Selection. Medical history also encourages and trains us to use an academic approach to our studies which thereby should be more precise, more meaningful, and more productive. Medical history should be enjoyable too, since that is a powerful stimulus to move forward, a fun thing to do.

The inspiring book that led to this series introduced us to clinical neurology, genetics, and the history of those with muscular dystrophy. Alan and Marcia Emery explored *The History of a Genetic Disease*, now often styled Meryon's disease rather than Duchenne muscular dystrophy. The first to describe a disease process is not necessarily the owner of the eponym but the Emerys are helping put that right for their subject, Edward Meryon.

This book on radiology takes us on a journey round the specialty. The volume could equally well have been described as a History of Medical Imaging since so much has happened here, as in almost every speciality in medicine, to improve our diagnosis and treatment of the ailments that can afflict us all. More always needs to be done, of course. Radiology has its own special place since at first it was concerned with producing pictures of broken bones and dislocated joints and then through various technical advances it has metamorphosed to a vast array of methods by which not only the anatomy but also the physiology of the body may be examined. Thus the authors describe the use of tomography, ultrasound, isotope studies, computed tomography, positron emission tomography, magnetic resonance imaging, and much else. These techniques enable doctors to see into the structure and workings of the body and, of course, have also been used in animal health, in the palaeoimaging of Egyptian mummies, in investigating the remains of sailors who died during the ill-fated Franklin Expedition of 1845–1848, and in many other circumstances.

Future volumes in this series of Oxford Medical Histories should take us to other aspects of our humanity, always leaving us with more questions than have been answered since each new discovery leads to more questions, exponential sets of issue for study, further thought, and an attempt to solve the big questions that surround our existence. Medicine is about people and so is history; the study of the combination of the duo can be very powerful. What do you think?

Christopher Gardner-Thorpe, MD, FRCP, FACP

Series Advisor, Oxford Medical Histories

Preface

The history of medicine from antiquity to the present day has been well chronicled in many notable scholarly texts. Radiology, which was founded in 1895 following Röntgen's discovery of X-rays, is a relatively new subspecialty of medicine and as such has often been neglected in medical historical books.

The history of the development of radiology, although a relatively new specialty, is an interesting story. Rapid advances in the 20th century in physics, chemistry, engineering, and computing enabled engineers, scientists, and doctors to collaborate and produce remarkable new machines, equipment, and techniques for investigating the human body, thus revolutionizing the science of medical imaging.

In this book the authors have tried to review the remarkable developments that occurred in the field of medical imaging since the discovery of X-rays and have tried to place the advances in not only a historical but also a cultural and social context. A work such as this is perhaps more notable for its omissions and it does not profess to be encyclopaedic. Great discoveries and inventions in medicine and science often result in accolades going to a few and these people are often said to have been privileged to stand on the shoulder of giants who have preceded them. A book like this would not have been possible without the help of previous scholars, libraries, and many learned institutions and their archives, journals, and collections which are acknowledged in the text and the references. We have attempted to tell the story of the last hundred years of radiology and hope the book will be of interest to a wide range of readers including doctors, scientists, medical physicists, radiographers, historians of medicine and science, as well as any interested lay person.

Most of the population will undergo some form of medical imaging during their lives. This book hopefully will serve to explain how current radiology developed from fairly humble beginnings to the modern, sophisticated, high-technology specialty of the 21st century.

In 1895 Sir William Osler, the distinguished physician and medical historian, wrote the following (taken from 'The Practical Values of Laveran's Discoveries') in the *Medical News, Philadelphia*:

> Even in well-known affections advances are made from time to time that render necessary a revision of our accumulated knowledge, a readjustment of old positions, a removal even of the old landmarks.[1]

Osler was then referring to the latest bacteriological discoveries. The remarks would have been just as prescient were he referring to Röntgen's discovery of X-rays which occurred soon after these words were written.

Reference

1. Osler, W. (1895). The practical value of Laveran's discoveries. *Medical News, Philadelphia*, 67, 561–564.

Contents

About the authors

Professor Adrian M.K. Thomas has been interested in history since his school days when he was taught by the author Glen Petrie. As an undergraduate at University College London he was privileged to study under Edwin Clarke, Jonathan Miller, and Bill Bynum. After entering radiology he was a founder member of the British Society for the History of Radiology. He has written three books on the history of radiology and has given many talks and presentations. He is the Honorary Librarian and Archivist of the British Institute of Radiology and the Clinical Director for Radiology for South London Healthcare NHS Trust. He is Chairman of the International Society for the History of Radiology and President of the British Society for the History of Medicine.

Dr Arpan K. Banerjee qualified in medicine from St Thomas's Hospital Medical School in London, UK. He was appointed a Consultant Radiologist at Birmingham Heartlands Hospital in 1995 and was also appointed an Honorary Clinical Senior Lecturer at the Birmingham Medical School that year.

From 2005 to 2007 he was President of the Radiology Section of the Royal Society of Medicine, London, where he continues to serve on the Council. In 2012 he was appointed Chairman of the British Society of the History of Radiology of which he is a founder member and council member. He is a founder member and Treasurer of the International Society for the History of Radiology (ISHRAD). In 2011 he was appointed a member of the scientific programme committee of the Royal College of Radiologists.

He is the author/co-author of six books including *Classic Papers in Modern Diagnostic Radiology* and the best-seller, *Radiology Made Easy*, three book chapters, and over 100 articles including over 50 peer-reviewed papers on medical, radiological, and medical historical topics.

Abbreviations

3-D	three-dimensional
BIR	British Institute of Radiology
BSIR	British Society of Interventional Radiology
CT	computed tomography
DHSS	Department of Health and Social Security
DSA	digital subtraction angiography
EMI	Electrical and Musical Industries
FNA	fine needle aspiration
ISRRT	International Society of Radiographers and Radiological Technicians
IT	information technology
IVU	intravenous urogram
LOCM	low-osmolar contrast media
MRI	magnetic resonance imaging
NMR	nuclear magnetic resonance
PACS	picture archiving and communication system
PET	positron emission tomography
PTC	percutaneous transhepatic cholangiography
RCR	Royal College of Radiologists
RIS	radiology information system
VS	Vascular Society of Great Britain and Ireland

Chapter 1

Wilhelm Röntgen and the discovery

The scientific background

It might naturally be expected that the beginning of a book on the history of radiology would commence with Wilhelm Röntgen's momentous discovery of X-rays in 1895, as has been recorded by Otto Glasser in his classic biography.[1] The story, however, does not begin there. The French scientist Louis Pasteur once said in a famous lecture delivered at the University of Lille in 1854 that 'chance prepares the favoured mind'.[2] Unfortunately the mind of Professor Arthur Willis Goodspeed, a professor of physics at the University of Pennsylvania, USA, was not favoured and today he is largely a forgotten figure. Arthur Goodspeed (1860–1943) was working with an English-born photographer, William N. Jennings (1860–1945), when on 22 February 1890 they produced, completely accidentally, a Röntgen ray picture, but were unable to work out what they had done and the significance of their findings were overlooked until 1895. Consequently they were not to share in the glories that were awarded to Wilhelm Röntgen and were destined for relative scientific obscurity. Goodspeed and Jennings used an induction coil and made a series of plates of coins and other small objects from the light generated from the sparks from the coil. The radiograph that was produced was in fact an X-ray accident and was not an intended consequence of their scientific endeavours. Only when Röntgen reported his findings in 1895 did the pair finally realize what they had overlooked.[3]

Nikola Tesla

In 1887, Nikola Tesla (1856–1943),[4] the Serbian electrical engineer and inventor, started experimenting with vacuum tubes with no electrodes.

Tesla, who had already invented the first loudspeaker and induction motor, had formed his own company in 1886, called the Tesla Electric Light & Manufacturing. In 1897 he invented the first alternating current induction motor and the following year developed the principles of the Tesla coil. The electrodeless tubes produced X-rays by virtue of the bremsstrahlung effect (or *braking radiation*). Tesla did not know then that this tube operated by emitting electrons from the single electrode through a combination of field electron emission and thermionic emission. Once released, the electrons were strongly repelled by the high electric field near the electrode during negative voltage peaks from the oscillating high-voltage output of the Tesla coil. X-rays were produced as the electrons collided with the glass envelope. Tesla, however, did not realize the significance of these rays, and he thought they were longitudinal waves. Although he observed as early as 1892 that skin could be damaged by the rays, he did not realize that it was the rays themselves that were harmful. Tesla, it is believed, even managed to obtain images of the bones of his hand but he did not widely disseminate his results. Although Tesla's contributions to the early discovery of X-rays is now largely forgotten, his inventive genius has left the world a large legacy of electrical engineering inventions and he is today remembered for the SI unit of magnetic flux density which has been named after him.

In the next 5 years between 1890 and 1895, European physicists including Heinrich Hertz (1857–1894), who was to go on to discover radio waves, were experimenting with cathode rays generated in Crookes tubes.[5] Hertz reported that X-rays could pass through a thin foil of aluminium within the tube and he believed that the cathode rays were waves rather than particles. Philip Lenard (1862–1947), who was one of Hertz's assistants and was to be awarded the Nobel Prize in Physics in 1905 for his work on cathode rays and radiation attenuation, modified the X-ray tube so that there was a thin aluminium foil window and discovered that rays could emerge through the window and be detected several inches away. These rays were called Lenard rays. Lenard had used a fluorescent substance unfit for X-rays and had used a sheet of metal which partly absorbed the X-rays rather than cardboard which was to be used in Röntgen's experiment. Much of the apparatus had its origin

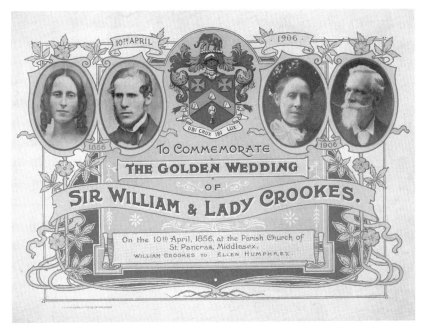

Fig. 1.1 Sir William Crookes and his wife, commemorating their golden wedding in 1906.

Reproduced with permission from the archive of the British Institute of Radiology.

in Britain. Michael Faraday (1791–1867) had discovered electromagnetism in the 1830s and this led to the introduction of the Rühmkorff induction coil and wet battery as a source of electricity. The main focus of the apparatus was the vacuum tube, which had been developed by the British scientist Sir William Crookes (1832–1919), who is illustrated on a card printed to celebrate his golden wedding anniversary (Figure 1.1).

Röntgen and the discovery

Lenard's new findings generated great interest among physicists and led to the seminal experiment of Wilhelm Conrad Röntgen on 8 November 1895, on a Friday afternoon. Röntgen, depicted in Figure 1.2 at the time of the discovery, was a relatively unknown 50-year-old professor of physics at the German University of Würzburg, and he essentially set out to conduct a similar experiment to what Professor Goodspeed had performed.[6] Röntgen, however, used a completely darkened room. He encased the

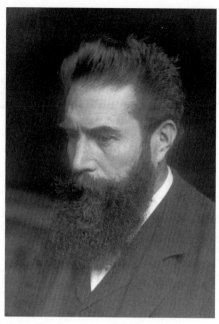

Fig. 1.2 Wilhelm Röntgen, the discoverer of X-rays.
Reproduced with permission from Deutsches Röntgen-Museum, Remscheid, Germany.

Crookes tube in a lightproof cardboard jacket and the barium platino-cyanide screen was only a few feet from the tube. As he conducted this experiment, Röntgen, to his surprise, found that the barium platino-cyanide screen lying on the bench was mysteriously lighting up. He continued to repeat his experiments, moving the screen further and further away from the tube. He realized that the fluorescence could not be due to cathode rays as these could not penetrate as far as 6 to 7 feet. Röntgen therefore concluded that this was a new kind of radiation, which was neither a visible light nor cathode rays, and that this new kind of radiation must be coming from the tube and causing the screen to fluoresce. The rest, of course, is history. Röntgen tentatively noted that the rays could pass through cardboard. A hand was placed between the Crookes tube and the fluorescent screen in one of his experiments and this, to Röntgen's amazement, revealed the bones of the hand clearly. A famous skiagram (the early name for a radiograph, deriving from the Greek word for shadow) of Röntgen's wife's hand was made on 22 December 1895, and Röntgen delivered his preliminary report entitled 'On a New Kind of Rays' to the Physical-Medical Society of Würzburg on 28 December 28 1895 for publication in the proceedings. Only the first page of his original manuscript survives; the rest was destroyed after his death as instructed in his will. On New Year's Day 1896 Röntgen sent some reports and sample X-ray prints to a wide range of eminent physicists including one in Vienna who passed it on to the editor of the Vienna newspaper, *Die Presse*. *Die Presse* reported the story on its front page on Sunday, 5 January 1896. The summary of this news was telegraphed to the *Daily Chronicle* in London and promptly to New York and suddenly news of this momentous discovery was disseminated throughout the world. In the USA, *The New York Sun* published a piece on 6 January 1896 to be followed by another article in *The New York Times* on 12 January 1896. Röntgen received congratulatory letters from many scientists including Albert Einstein, Marie Curie, Lord Kelvin, and Thomas Edison.

In the well-known interview with Röntgen by the American H.J.W. Dam, published by *Pearson's Magazine* in 1896, the following was recorded:

"What was the date?"

"The 8th of November."

"And what was the discovery?"

"I was working with a Crookes tube covered by a shield of black cardboard. A piece of barium platino-cyanide paper lay on the bench there. I had been passing a current through the tube, and I noticed a peculiar black line across the paper."

"What of that?"

"The effect was one which could only be produced in ordinary parlance by the passage of light. No light could come from the tube, because the shield which covered it was impervious to any light known, even the electric arc."

"And what did you think?"

"I did not think, I investigated. I assumed that the effect must come from the tube since its character indicated that it could come from nowhere else. I tested it. In a few moments there was no doubt about it. Rays were coming from the tube, which had a luminescent effect upon the paper. I tried it successfully at greater and greater distances, even at two metres. It seemed at first a new kind of invisible light. It was clearly something new, something unrecorded."

"Is it light?"

"No."

"Is it electricity?"

"Not in any known form."

"What is it?"
"I don't know."[7]

(Reproduced from H.J.W Dam, A Wizard of Today,
Pearson's Magazine, *1*, pp. 413–419, Copyright © 1896)

And so Dam went away having recorded in his interview that the now famous discoverer of the X-rays was entirely ignorant as to the nature of their essence.[7]

Early reception of the discovery

In the UK, news of the discovery was printed in *The Manchester Guardian* on 7 January and also in the London *Evening Standard* on 7 and 8 January 1896.[8] The prestigious science journal *Nature* on 16 January was, however, more reserved about the discovery. The translation of the article 'On a New Kind of Rays' was printed in the 23 January issue of *Nature*, the translation being sent by Professor Arthur Schuster of Manchester although it is claimed that the translation was probably made by his assistant, Arthur Stanton. The leading medical journal *The Lancet* published an editorial entitled 'A Search Light of Photography' and was somewhat sceptical of the discovery. It was left to the *British Medical Journal* to champion Röntgen's discovery in the UK. The journal commissioned a Mr Sidney Rowland (1872–1917), who was a young medical graduate from St Bartholomew's Hospital in London, to write articles on this new form of photography. Sidney Rowland's uncle, Ernest Hart, happened to be the editor of the journal and whilst this was a good example of nepotism, the young Rowland did an excellent job. Sidney Rowland became a champion of X-rays and demonstrated X-rays at the Medical Society of London. Figure 1.3 shows Sidney Rowland in 1896—note the absence of protection around the Crookes tube. It is ironic that although Sidney Rowland did much to publicize X-rays, his real passion was bacteriology and he went to work for the Lister Institute in London. He was to eventually die of cerebrospinal fever in 1917 in France, where he was in charge of a bacteriological laboratory during the First World War.

By early 1896, news had travelled fast around the world and several British pioneers were experimenting with the technique of X-rays.

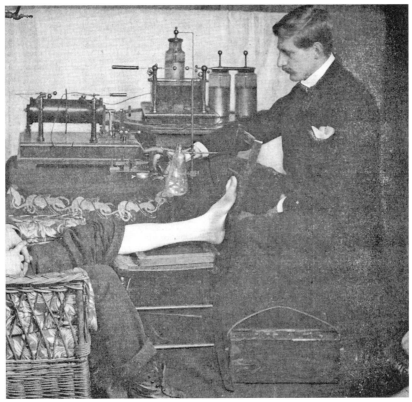

Fig. 1.3 Sidney Rowland, the editor of the first ever journal of radiology.

Early pioneers included John Francis Hall-Edwards (1858–1926) in Birmingham who with J.R. Ratcliffe produced radiographs within only a few days of the discovery. In Sheffield, Professor Hicks produced early radiographs of two patients with needles in soft tissues localized by the X-ray method and the cases were reported in the *British Medical Journal*. In Bristol, a surgeon, Charles Morton, produced excellent radiographs of a cadaveric foot into which he had inserted a needle. Alan A. Campbell Swinton (1863–1930), a self-taught non-medical experimenter with an interest in photography, electricity, and experimentation (later to become a Fellow of the Royal Society), delivered a lecture to the Royal Photographic Society on 11 February 1896 entitled 'A New Shadow Photography' and gave the first public demonstration of the art of radiography in England. Swinton said that the photographs were of the nature of shadows, though shadows produced by rays which are not luminous. Lecture demonstrations continued unabated and early contributions to the literature included one of the earliest textbooks entitled *Practical Radiography*, written by A.W. Isenthal and H. Snowden Ward (Isenthal was an early supporter and council member of the Röntgen Society and an early supplier of X-ray equipment). Figure 1.4 illustrates the blurred images that were obtained using the early apparatus.

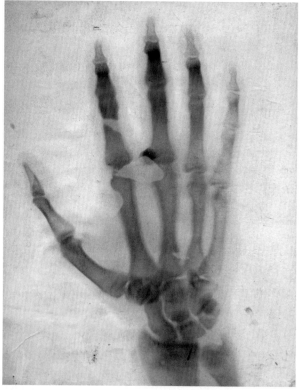

Fig. 1.4 Hand of the pioneer radiologist Sebastian Gilbert Scott taken in 1897. The central dark shadow is a bullet.

Image donated by the Scott family. Reproduced courtesy of Dr Adrian M.K. Thomas.

The Nobel Prize

Röntgen was honoured with the first Nobel Prize in Physics, awarded in 1901. The citation read 'The Academy has awarded Professor Röntgen of Munich the Nobel Prize for Physics on the grounds of discovery, the name of which will always be linked with him as Röntgen rays or as he calls them himself X-rays…From the properties associated with Röntgen rays, only those are considered that contribute to the far reaching applications these rays have found in medical practice.'[9] The Nobel Prize medal and the first page of his famous manuscript can be seen today at the Deutsche Röntgen Museum in Remscheid, Germany, in the museum which is devoted to Röntgen, the discovery of X-rays, and their subsequent application in medical science.

References

1. **Glasser, O.** (1934). *William Conrad Röntgen and the Early History of the Roentgen Rays*. Springfield, IL: Charles C. Thomas.
2. **Vallery-Radot, R.** (1915). *The Life of Pasteur*. New York, NY: Doubleday.
3. **Brecher, E. and Brecher, R.** (1969). *The Rays—History of Radiology in the United States and Canada*. Baltimore, MD: Williams and Wilkins.
4. **Cheney, M. and Uth, R.** (1999). *Tesla, Master of Lightning*. New York, NY: Fall River Press.
5. **Glasser, O.** (1945). Scientific forefathers of Roentgen. *American Journal of Roentgenology, 54*, 545–546.
6. **Claxton, K.P.** (1970). *Wilhelm Roentgen*. Geneva: Edito-service SA.
7. **Dam, H.J.W.** (1896). A wizard of today. *Pearson's Magazine, 1*, 413–419.
8. **Thomas, A.M.K. and Guy, J.M.** (1995). The early reception of Röntgen's discovery in the United Kingdom. In Thomas, A.M.K., Isherwood, I., and Wells, P.N.T. (Eds), *The Invisible Light. 100 Years of Medical Radiology*, PP. 7–12. Oxford: Blackwell Science.
9. *Nobel Lectures, Physics 1901–1921*. (1967). Amsterdam: Elsevier.

Chapter 2

Early radiology

The importance of the X-ray machine to the general public is shown by the fact that in 2009 it won the Science Museum's Centenary Award. The modern Science Museum in London was founded in 1909 and as part of its centenary celebrations it held a public vote on the top ten objects in the museum. One of the icons is the Russell Reynolds X-ray apparatus, which is on display in their 'Making of the Modern World' gallery. In January 1896, as a schoolboy, Russell Reynolds (1880–1964) used an early Watson gas X-ray tube mounted on a retort stand similar to the one illustrated to demonstrate Röntgen's discovery (Figure 2.1). Nearly 50,000 people voted in the poll, and they voted overwhelmingly for the discoveries that have transformed the way we look at our bodies and ourselves. The X-ray machine took the top place, followed by penicillin and then the DNA double helix. We should also reflect on the fact that without X-ray crystallography the discovery of the structure of DNA (which took third place in the vote) would not have happened.

Early radiology was both difficult and dangerous.[1] There was no radiation protection of the X-ray tube or indeed any electrical protection of the apparatus. There were a number of dangers that were intrinsic to early radiology, and these included the dangers of overexposure to radiation, the presence of high-tension cables, and also the chemicals involved in photographic wet processing. It was not until the 1930s that shockproof apparatus became generally available. There is an account of the inquest of a nurse at Wimbledon Hospital in the 1930s who was killed by an electrical shock after being repeatedly warned by the radiographer to keep away from the mobile ward apparatus when an exposure was being made. The unfortunate nurse touched the radiographic apparatus as the exposure was being made and received a fatal shock.

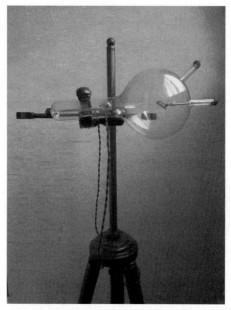

Fig. 2.1 An early gas (ion) X-ray tube mounted on a wooden stand.
Image courtesy of Dr Adrian M.K. Thomas.

Ernest Wilson (1871–1911)

The story of Ernest Wilson illustrates the dangers that beset the pioneers. Ernest Wilson was for some years a lay assistant (radiographer) at the Electrotherapeutic Department at the London Hospital (now the Royal London Hospital), having joined the department in 1899. Initially all his work involved the use of the fluorescent screen, and this was carried out with no protection. Wilson held a fluorescent screen for many hours each day, exposing his hands in particular to the full effect of the rays. He was 'not of a robust type' and had previously suffered from tuberculosis of his neck glands. Within a few months of his starting to work with X-rays his hands showed evidence of X-ray injury (radiation dermatitis) and by 1900 he had developed whitlows at the base of the nails. Initially these were treated by 'scraping and fomenting'. A series of amputations of the right middle finger were performed, starting in June 1904; these never healed well and there followed chronic suppuration. He took a poignant series of radiographs of his hands demonstrating the progressive changes (Figure 2.2). By June 1910 the stump was very painful and swollen and a further amputation was performed. The specimen showed evidence of epithelioma, which was spreading along the bone. At this period the possibility of the development of epithelioma in such cases was only just being realized. A final amputation of the

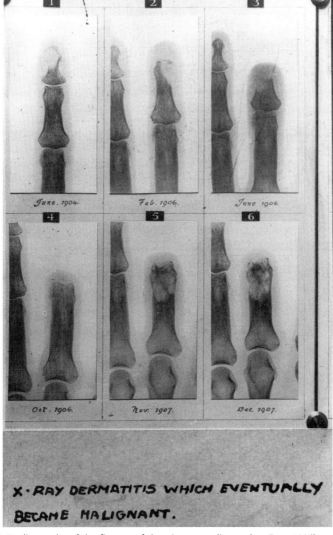

Fig. 2.2 Radiographs of the fingers of the pioneer radiographer Ernest Wilson showing progressive bony loss secondary to radiation injury.

Image donated by the Scott Family. Reproduced courtesy of Dr Adrian M.K. Thomas.

finger was soon followed by axillary lymphadenopathy with secondary deposits and he died on 1 March 1911 at the age of 40. As Ernest Wilson put it himself, he was not a martyr to science but a victim since a martyr knows what to expect. His name was one of the original 169 names of X-ray and radium martyrs recorded on the memorial in the grounds of St George's Hospital, Hamburg.

It was on 4 April 1936 that a memorial to the X-ray martyrs of the world was erected in the grounds of St George's Hospital in Hamburg. The monument is still standing and may be visited. These early X-ray and radium workers suffered greatly from radiation injuries and pre-mature death in the period prior to the understanding of the need for radiation protection and safe handling of radiation sources. In particular, there was little awareness of the cumulative nature of exposure. It was believed that if a radiation worker showed signs of overexposure then what was needed was a period of rest and recuperation. Once the worker had recovered then he or she could safely return to work. This is not the case and radiation doses are cumulative.

Corporal Edward Wallwork RAMC and radiation risks

Unfortunately there were many of the early generation of X-ray workers who suffered injuries from radiation. The illustration (Figure 2.3) shows a wristwatch presented to Corporal Edward Wallwork RAMC by Doctors Ironside Bruce (1879–1921), Stanley Melville (1867–1934), and George Harrison Orton (1873–1947). The presentation of the watch was as a token of appreciation for his work in the X-ray department of the King George Hospital in London from 1915 to 1919. The watch measures 3cm and is engraved on the back. Edward Wallwork was from the Manchester area. All of the three doctors suffered from radiation-induced disease and their names are recorded on the X-ray martyrs' memorial in the grounds of St George's Hospital in Hamburg. Ironside Bruce was on the staff of Charing Cross Hospital and the Hospital for Sick Children in Great Ormond Street. Ironside Bruce was very talented and published widely and his well-known book *A System of Radiology: with an Atlas of the Normal* came out in 1907. The British radiological world was shocked when Bruce died of radiation-induced

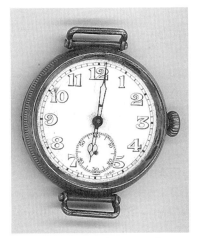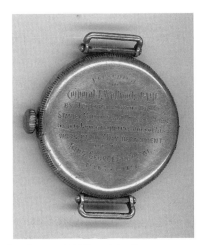

Fig. 2.3 The engraved wristwatch presented to Corporal Wallwork by three radiologists who all became radiation martyrs.

Reproduced with permission from the archive of the British Institute of Radiology.

aplastic anaemia in 1921 at the young age of 42. The outcry resulting from his death resulted in the formation of a national radiation protection committee. George Harrison Orton was a pioneer of radiotherapy and was in charge of the X-ray department at St Mary's Hospital in London. George Orton was regarded as the last martyr pioneer of radiology. Stanley Melville worked at St George's Hospital in London and was the President of the British Institute of Radiology in 1934. Both Orton and Melville served periods as co-secretary with Sidney Russ of the newly formed and influential British 'X-ray and Radium Protection Committee'. Concerns about the safety of radiation continue to this day and medical radiation is now a significant proportion of the population's exposure to radiation.

The United Nations was concerned about the responsibilities of the medical profession to limit the medical use of ionizing radiation and issued a statement in June 1957 that is still relevant today. In 1956 the British government under the chairmanship of Lord Adrian had set up a committee on radiation hazards to patients and in June 1957 Adrian was asking for the help and assistance of radiologists through the pages of the *British Journal of Radiology*. Concerns about medical radiation became more significant as the 1950s progressed in the period after Hiroshima and Nagasaki when public concern about radiation was heightened. In the UK in August 1957 Sir Stanford Cade reviewed radiation-induced cancer in humans and G.M. Ardran advised the radiological community on dose reduction in diagnostic radiology and how it might be achieved. G.M. Ardran and H.E. Crooks also reviewed doses from dental radiography and the effect of radiographic techniques in September 1959. The Presidential Address by L.F. Lamerton for 1958 to the British Institute of Radiology examined the clinical and experimental data for the risks to the individual of small doses of radiation and arguments over the importance of small doses of radiation continue to this day. Basically, is there a threshold for the effects of radiation or is all radiation harmful? This question is still controversial. In April 1959, A.G.S. Cooper and A.W. Steinbeck from Australia reported a case of leukaemia developing in a 3-year-old child following irradiation whilst *in utero*, and in an adult man following spinal irradiation for ankylosing spondylitis. Concerns about the effects of antenatal radiography had been raised by the Oxford epidemiologist Alice Stewart in 1956. By the 1930s many obstetricians were recommending routing prenatal radiography and the risk of radiation to mother and fetus were generally minimized by the medical profession. It was Alice Stewart[2] who correlated cancer deaths in children under the age of 15 to the mother being exposed to radiography in pregnancy. Stewart was investigating the epidemiology of childhood leukaemia, which in 1951 was rising in frequency and a 'leukaemia epidemic' was being talked about. Alice Stewart emphasized the obvious fact that life begins at conception and not at birth, and she therefore asked mothers about what happened during their pregnancy, such as 'Did you have any illnesses in pregnancy?' and 'Were you X-rayed?'.[2] This research was undertaken at the height of the 'Cold War' at a time of increasing concerns about radiation. The Campaign for Nuclear Disarmament was formed in 1958, which was the same year that Alice Stewart's full study was published. In that year Linus Pauling (the winner of the 1954 Nobel Prize for Chemistry) suggested that nuclear fallout from nuclear testing could have effects on the fetus and result in injury, and for his pains Pauling had to appear before the House of Un-American Activities (HUAC) and it was made difficult for him at Cal Tech, precipitating his resignation. In spite of the evidence there was resistance in the medical profession to a change in practice and whilst there was some fall off in requests for radiography in pregnancy it was not until 1980 that major American medical groups ceased to recommend the practice.

In 1961 the Medical Research Council in the UK reported on the hazards of radiation in their second report on the topic and the important Adrian Committee on Radiological Hazards to Patients also reported. The reports were very influential and became 'required reading for all radiologists'. Lord Adrian gave the opening address to the Annual UK Radiology Congress in 1961 and his views on the hazards of radiation remain relevant to this day. The hazards of medical radiation were now being taken seriously and efforts to reduce doses to patients and operators were made in both diagnostic radiology and radiotherapy and numerous publications appeared. By 1969 Jennifer Matthews from Sheffield repeated a survey of radiation hazards in diagnostic radiology. She found that whilst the staff were aware of radiation risks and used gonadal shields, the numbers of patients radiographed were continuing to rise. This remains true with yearly increases in the use of computed tomography (CT) scanning. However, the risks of any technique have to be balanced against the benefits and not having the CT scan may be more harmful than having the test.

The acronym ALARA stands for 'as low as reasonably achievable' and this idea started to develop in the 1950s with the concerns about radiation exposure. In the 1960s the Atomic Energy Commission, required that human exposures be kept 'as low as practicable' (ALAP). ALARA was recognized at this time, although there was more concern about controlling radiation exposures to within the dose limits, rather than reducing them to below the limits. Concerns ware also present in the 1970s with the recognition of the development of solid tumours in the Japanese survivors of the atomic bombs from the Second World War and in patients receiving radiotherapy. Whilst tumours may develop with high doses of radiation the effects of small doses are less certain, hence the need to keep doses ALARA, although economic and social factors need to be taken into consideration. A balance needs to be made between the clinical value of an examination and the radiation dose received. For example, a radiograph of a foot to diagnose a fracture or arthritis is reasonable. Using radiology to fit shoes in the Pedoscope that was popular in the 1950s and earlier is not.

Early pioneers

Charles Thurstan Holland (1863–1941)[3] (Figure 2.4) was a major figure in early radiology both in the UK and worldwide. Holland worked as a general practitioner in Liverpool from 1889 and following the discovery of X-rays he was approached by Robert Jones (1857–1933) who was a pioneer orthopaedic surgeon. As Holland recollected, 'In the beginning of 1896 Robert Jones visualized some of the possibilities of radiography in respect to his own work'.[3] His first radiograph was made on 29 May 1896 and was 'My first X-ray. My own hand'. This involved a 2-minute exposure using a 3-inch coil and five Grove cells. He took a total of 261 plates in 1896. Holland radiographed many conditions including foreign bodies, arthritis, fractures, a stillborn fetus (Figure 2.5), 'mummy bird', fish to show bones, and a series of hands to demonstrate bone growth. Whilst his images may look basic today the difficulties that he overcame and the skills that he showed cannot be overemphasized. What is remarkable about the pioneers is how many future developments were anticipated. As Holland recalled, 'There were no X-ray departments in any of the hospitals. There were no experts. There was no literature. No one knew anything about radiographs of the normal, to say nothing of the abnormal'.[3] Writing in 1938, R.E. Roberts was able to say that 'In spite of the inadequate apparatus which was available, and of the lengthy exposures required, some of Holland's early radiographs of small parts compare very favourably with many of those seen nowadays, taken with much more costly equipment'.[3]

Thurstan Holland was President of the Röntgen Society (1904–1905) and in 1925 was President of the First International Congress of Radiology, held in London. It is now quite difficult to put ourselves into the mind-set of the pioneers in the 1890s. There was a confidence that we now lack. In his presidential address to the Liverpool and Literary

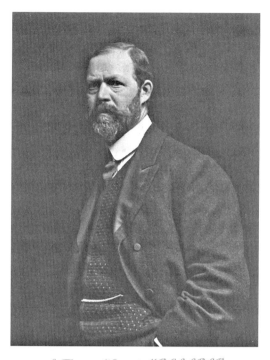

C. Thurstan Holland, M.R.C.S., L.R.C.P.
President of the Röntgen Society 1904-1905.

Fig. 2.4 The pioneer Liverpool radiologist Dr Charles Thurstan Holland as President of the Röntgen Society, 1904.

Reproduced with permission from the archive of the British Institute of Radiology.

Society in October 1896 Holland could explain that 'this 19th century of ours is the most wonderful that the world has ever seen' and 'In the case of operative we have almost reached the acme of this art. It is difficult to see in what way it can make any further great advances'.[4] How wrong he was and the speciality of radiology to which he was to contribute so much was to transform surgical practice.

A letter sent by Patrick Heron Watson of Charlotte Square in Edinburgh to Dawson Turner (1857–1928), the pioneer Edinburgh radiologist at George Square, dated 17 February 1896 (Figure 2.6), enclosed a cheque for five guineas (£5.25) as payment for the 'photoprinting of the hand with Enchondromata as illustrating the Röntgen process'. Five guineas was a considerable sum of money in 1896. This is possibly the

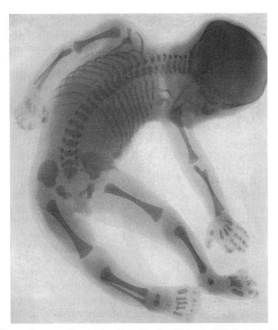

Fig. 2.5 A stillborn fetus radiographed by Charles Thurstan Holland in 1896.

Reproduced with permission from C. Thurstan Holland, X Rays in 1896, *British Journal of Radiology*, Vol. *11*, No. 121, pp. 1–24, Copyright © 1938 British Institute of Radiology, DOI: 10.1259/0007-1285-11-121-1. Image kindly supplied by the archive of the British Institute of Radiology.

earliest account of a payment for radiological services and is dated less than 4 months after the discovery of X-rays. Dawson Turner was the first doctor to provide radiological services to the Edinburgh Royal Infirmary. Sadly Dawson Turner had to retire early due to the injurious effects of radiation and his name is one of three from Edinburgh to be listed on the Martyrs' Memorial at Hamburg.

Defining the normal

Defining what is normal might seem straightforward; however, it is actually quite difficult. The new rays gave us a different view of the body and interpretation of the shadows had to be made with care and, as Charles Thurstan Holland, the pioneer radiologist from Liverpool said, there were no experts, no literature, and no knowledge of the normal, to say nothing of the abnormal. In defining normal appearances

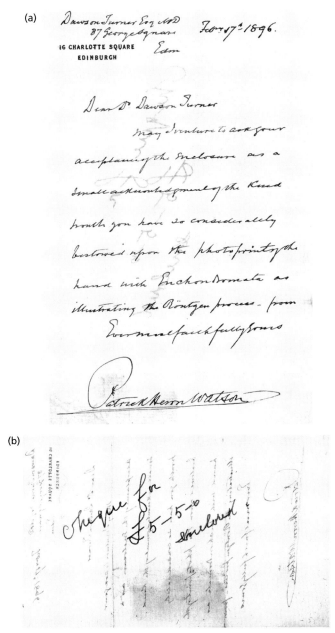

Fig. 2.6 A letter sent by Patrick Heron Watson of Charlotte Square in Edinburgh to Dawson Turner enclosing a cheque for five guineas as payment for radiological services. Dated 17 February 1896 it may be the earliest financial transaction radiological services in existence.

Image courtesy of Dr Adrian M.K. Thomas.

in radiography the work of Alban Köhler from Germany and Sebastian Gilbert Scott from England is important.

In the case of the Nelson incident (described later), the radiological abnormality was obvious. However, other abnormalities that are of forensic importance are considerably subtler. The shadows cast by the new rays discovered by Röntgen could often be confusing and until the normal was defined the medico-legal use of radiographs as evidence could only be limited.[5] The question, though, as to what is normal is not as simple as it might first appear. Traditional anatomy had been learnt in the dissecting room or in the operating theatre and the new living anatomy shown on radiographs required a new appreciation and understanding of anatomy and its many variations. Since earliest times variations from normality had been recognized, particularly in the animal kingdom. Before radiography the knowledge of human congenital anomalies, apart from gross and visible anomalies, was limited to those found by anatomists at dissection. If the nature of normality is not appreciated in clinical practice there is a danger of medical intervention for non-existent conditions. For example, a lack of understanding of the normal anatomy and physiology as shown on radiography led to 'fantasy surgery' for dropped organs (visceroptosis and floating kidneys) and chronic intestinal stasis.[6] The position of a kidney lying down is different from that standing up and both are normal. There is also a wide variation in the shape and position of the stomach and when standing up part of the stomach may lie in the pelvis. Ann Dally has reviewed the story of surgery for 'displaced' organs and for chronic intestinal stasis as a cause for a large variety of symptoms. The subject of chronic intestinal stasis was reviewed by Alfred Jordan in 1923 and he called it Arbuthnot Lane's disease, dedicating the book to him as 'The Father of Stasis'. Jordan provided the radiological evidence for Lane's surgical practice and his book is full of examples of colonic and duodenal stasis. It is easy to be critical of those in the past while being blind to our own failings. The significance of the abnormalities that we find on modern medical imaging is often not obvious, particularly on magnetic resonance imaging (MRI). More tests are being performed on patients and an increasing number of coincidental abnormalities are found of uncertain significance to the patient's presenting complaint. The term 'Ulysses syndrome' has been coined for the practice of intensive investigation of coincidental abnormalities that are not related to the patient's primary condition. Whilst the adventures of Ulysses as described in *The Odyssey* by Homer are interesting, his aim was to return home to his wife.

Alban Köhler (1874–1947)

The majority of congenital variations were undiscovered before the advent of modern medical imaging and the numbers of such variations increase as imaging becomes more sophisticated. It was largely due to the work of Köhler (1874–1947) of Wiesbaden in Germany that these variations of anatomy were first described. Köhler is best remembered today for his description of avascular necrosis of the tarsal navicular bone, which he described in 1908. Köhler was a founder member of the German Röntgen Society and became its president in 1912. The *Lexikon der Grenzen der Normalen und der Anfänge des Pathologischen im Röntgenbilde*[7] was published by Köhler in 1910 and went through a number of German editions and received the highest Röntgen award in Germany, the 'Rieder Gold Medal'. The book was enormously influential and became an immediate classic. Instead of reproducing radiographs, the book was illustrated using line drawings, and the illustration shown is of congenital abnormalities of the patellae (Figure 2.7). The book was translated into English in 1931, appearing as *Röntgenology: The Borderlands of the Normal and Early Pathological in the Skiagram*,[8] with a second edition appearing in 1935. In the preface to the second English edition, the great American radiologist James T. Case indicated the usefulness of the book 'to physicians and lawyers whose work brings them in contact with problems on legal medicine'.[9] Case wrote that 'how many foolish actions would be avoided and unjust decisions righted by a sufficient dissemination of the knowledge of developmental appearances in the radiogram'.[9] He then described a ridiculous damage suit over an alleged fracture of the spine, allowed as a just claim in a high court of law. The deciding testimony was that of a surgeon who declared the radiograph clearly demonstrated a fracture, whereas in reality it was a long-standing hypertrophic osteoarthritis with huge osteophytes

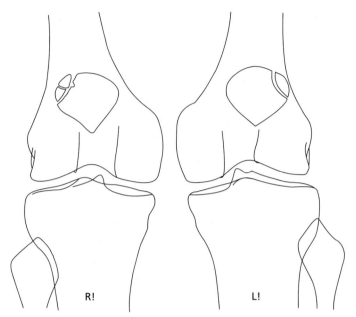

Fig. 2.7 Congenital abnormalities for the knees (bipartite patellae) as illustrated by Alban Köhler in 1910.

Originally published in Köhler, A., *Lexikon der Grenzen des Normalen und der Anfänge des Pathologischen im Röntgenbilde*, Lucas Gräfe & Sillem, Hamburg, Germany, Copyright © 1910. Image courtesy of Dr Adrian M.K. Thomas.

almost uniting the lumbar vertebrae into one bony mass; and what the surgeon interpreted as a fracture was in reality only a small island of calcification just separating two of the opposing bony outgrowths. In this instance, faulty evidence based on ignorance led to a serious miscarriage of justice. The radiological community therefore owes a huge debt to the pioneer work of Alban Köhler.

Sebastian Gilbert Scott

Dr Sebastian Gilbert Scott was the director of the radiological department of the London Hospital and was interested in medical jurisprudence and in skeletal variations. His influential book *Radiology in Relation to Medical Jurisprudence* was published in 1931.[10] By the 1930s many claims for compensation were being made in the UK at common law or under the Employer's Liability and Workmen's Compensation

Acts of 1905 and 1925. Scott held the view that large sums were being paid out each year that would not have been awarded if there were more awareness of skeletal variations and other conditions that made accurate diagnosis difficult, even for experienced radiologists. By the 1930s evidence of bone injury in medico-legal cases was almost entirely dependent on the radiographic appearances and the evidence of the radiologist was frequently the decisive factor in such cases. The misinterpretation of a supernumerary ossicle as a fracture would result in the payment of a large sum in compensation. The correct interpretation of the radiograph was therefore essential and the radiologist had to be familiar with the skeletal variations that may simulate a fracture. Scott pointed out that improvements in radiographic technique, instead of making that task easier, had made interpretation more difficult because of the increased detail that was then attainable. This trend has continued to contemporary times. Modern MRI and CT scans show much more detail than with earlier generations of scanners and the possibility of an improper interpretation increases with the complexity of the system.

In the UK in 1927 there were a total of 458,419 accidents to workmen that involved payments under the Workmen's Compensation Act with a total of £12 million.[10] Scott describe the case of a man with a congenital anomaly of the clavicle who had a series of imaginary accidents and had been able to successfully make a series of bogus claims to insurance companies.

In the 1930s the Medical Defence Union in the UK, which provided professional insurance for medical practitioners in cases of medical negligence, advised its members that in every case of fracture or suspected fracture a radiograph should be obtained. If the patient objected to a radiograph being obtained, then such a refusal should be obtained in writing. If this were not obtained than the Medical Defence Union might refuse to defend the case.

Scott emphasized the need for specialist interpretation of radiographs since there were many pitfalls and difficulties in image interpretation and these were illustrated in his book. Adequate training in image interpretation was therefore essential. By the 1920s there had been considerable developments in radiology and it was becoming recognized as a distinct medical speciality. The radiologist was defined as a qualified doctor with specialized training and in possession of a recognized qualification. The first qualification in the UK, and probably the world, was the Diploma in Medical Radiology and Electrology (DMRE), which was awarded by the University of Cambridge from 1922.

Scott also recommended the use of standard views in radiography. Standard views made image interpretation easier and facilitated comparison between radiographs taken by different radiologists and departments. If radiographs were not taken in standard positions then accurate comparison was made difficult. In the 1920s and 1930s standard radiographic views were developed, culminating in the publication of *Positioning in Radiography* by Kathleen C. Clark in 1929. The adequate identification of the radiograph was essential to avoid dispute and as adhesive labels were not acceptable the side marker was applied using a lead letter placed on the film before exposure.

Scott discussed in detail aspects of medico-legal work for radiologists. The radiographic report for medico-legal cases required special care in writing. Each statement in the report should be carefully considered with ambiguity avoided. The radiologist should keep strictly to the radiographic findings and not stray beyond his area of expertise. Radiographic imaging is an integral part of the medical process and provides a permanent record of the patient's condition.

The work of the pioneers Alban Köhler and Sebastian Gilbert Scott has been continued by Theodore Keats from Charlottesville, Virginia. His well-known *Atlas of Normal Roentgen Variants That May Simulate Disease* first appeared in 1973 and is currently in its ninth edition, and is a modern classic.[11] Its presence in most if not all radiology departments is witness to its value.

Kathleen Clark (1898–1968) and radiographic standardization

In the 1930s there was a gradual standardization of radiographic projections, which was to culminate in the publication of *Positioning in Radiography* by Kathleen C. Clark in January 1939. The book is a radiographic classic and remains in print to this day.

The Society of Radiographers had been set up in 1920. Letters had been written from the new society to non-medical assistants in the various X-ray departments in the UK inviting applications for membership. Those who been in active practice for over 10 years were given membership without examination; however, all other applicants had to take a new examination. The first regular group of students was entered for examination in January 1922. There were 45 students of which 20 passed and were duly awarded the certificate of the Society (the MSR). Miss K.C. Clark had completed her training course at Guy's Hospital in London in 1921 and she passed this first ever qualifying examination held by the Society of Radiographers. She worked initially at the Princess Mary's Hospital in Margate before moving to the Royal Northern Hospital in North London.

Clark was very aware of the lack of adequate training for radiographers and so she founded a school of radiography at the Royal Northern Hospital. This school became a model for schools of radiography elsewhere in the world. In 1935 she became co-founder and principal of the Ilford Radiographic Department at Tavistock House in London where she was involved in instruction and research into radiography and medical photography. Under her guidance the department developed a worldwide reputation. She was president of the Society of Radiographers from 1935 to 1937 (and also the first woman president) and is shown wearing the chain of office in Figure 2.8.

The first edition of her classic book *Positioning in Radiography* was published in 1939.[12] The book is the standard work of reference for radiographers and has been through many editions. Many radiographers will have heard of 'Kitty Clark' and have used the textbook.

Positioning in Radiography is a very important book for several reasons. Firstly, it standardized the radiographic projections and so similar projections were made in all hospitals. Clark was keen to standardize both the radiographic positioning and the exposure values. Secondly, the book is very artistic. The illustrations do not come across as cold and entirely objective scientific images. It is therefore not surprising to read that the artist Francis Bacon acknowledged *Positioning in*

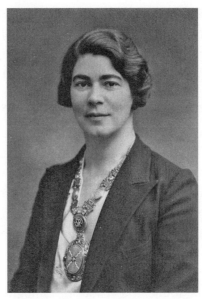

Fig. 2.8 Miss Kathleen Clark, president of the Society of Radiographers, 1935–1937. Reproduced with permission from the Society and College of Radiographers.

Radiography as a crucial source and it was his favourite medical textbook. Lawrence Gowling indicated that Bacon repeatedly borrowed from the photographs in the book for his work and pages torn out of the book were found in his studio. The images of the body that Francis Bacon painted have an almost radiographic quality and there is the impression that multiple layers of the body are seen at the same time and that one is not just looking at the skin surface.

K.C. Clark was awarded the MBE in 1945 for her services to radiography, particularly for her work on mass miniature radiography of the chest. She was committed to fostering cooperation and contact between radiographers throughout the world and was a driving spirit behind the formation of the International Society of Radiographers and Radiological Technicians (ISRRT). The photograph from 1964 (Figure 2.9) shows three important radiographers, K.C. Clark, E.R. Hutchinson, and Marion Frank. Ernest Ray 'Hutch' Hutchinson was president of the Society of Radiographers from 1959–1960 and Miss Marion Frank from 1967–1968. Kathleen Clark is on their right. All

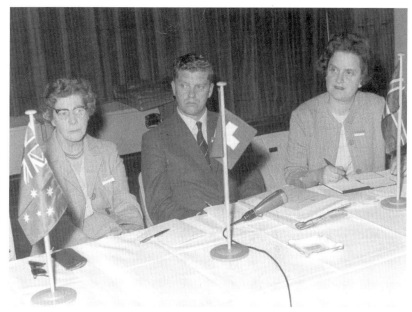

Fig. 2.9 Three radiographers: Kathleen Clark, Ernest Hutchinson, and Marion Frank.
Image donated by Kathleen Clark. Reproduced courtesy of Dr Adrian M.K. Thomas.

three were committed to international radiography and were involved in the formation of the ISRRT. The ISRRT is an organization composed of 71 national radiographic societies from 68 countries and now representing more than 200,000 radiographers and radiological technologists. K.C. Clark remained as principal at Ilford until 1958 and as consultant in radiography until 1964.

British Authors

A profession is defined by a number of parameters, one of which includes having a literature. One of the most significant events of the 1930s was the publication of *A Text-Book of X-ray Diagnosis by British Authors*, the highly influential multiauthor textbook covering all aspects of medical imaging. Diagnostic radiology came of age in this decade and this book celebrated the knowledge that had been obtained in the previous 40 years. The editors were Ernest W. Twining, C. Cochrane Shanks, and Peter Kerley, and the first edition was published in 1938. The book was expensive and volume 1 alone cost 50 shillings (£2.50). The standard that was set was quite outstanding and no other country produced anything that could compare, either in printing or in the illustrations. The book was required reading for generations of radiologists studying for examinations. It was the view of the radiologist Bill Park that during the lifetime of this book, the role of the radiologist advanced from a type of 'aircraft spotter' to that of an established clinical diagnostician. It was partly due to the contribution of this book that there was this fundamental change in attitudes. The final edition of the book was the fourth edition (edited by Cochrane Shanks and Peter Kerley following the untimely death of Ernest Twining) with volume 6 appearing in 1974. In our world now dominated by cross-sectional imaging we should remember those who worked with X-rays alone and who laid the foundations of the specialty of radiology. As a chest radiologist, Peter Kerley would have found MRI and CT quite fascinating in the details that they reveal of anatomy and pathology in the chest.

Early departments

John Macintyre and the Glasgow Royal Infirmary

John Macintyre (1857–1928)[12] was born in Glasgow and graduated in 1882 from the University of Glasgow. In 1885 he was appointed as medical electrician to the Glasgow Royal Infirmary and as assistant surgeon in 1886 with an interest in diseases of the ears, nose, and throat. After the discovery of X-rays in 1895, Röntgen sent a copy of his paper to various scientists around the world, including Lord Kelvin (1824–1907) who was one of the most famous physicists of that period. Kelvin passed the paper to J.T. Bottomley who contacted Macintyre and they then both worked together on demonstrating the new discovery. The letter that Lord Kelvin wrote to Röntgen on 17 January 1896 is preserved in the Deutsche Röntgen Museum (Figure 2.10); however, the radiographs that Röntgen had sent to Kelvin have been lost. In January 1896 Macintyre lectured at the University of Glasgow on 'The New Light—X-rays' and then on 15 February 1896, Bottomley, Lord Blythswood, and John Macintyre gave a presentation to the Philosophical Society of Glasgow.

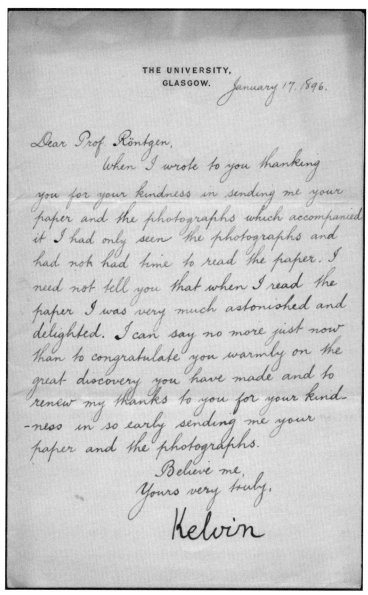

THE UNIVERSITY,
GLASGOW. *January 17, 1896.*

Dear Prof. Röntgen,

When I wrote to you thanking you for your kindness in sending me your paper and the photographs which accompanied it I had only seen the photographs and had not had time to read the paper. I need not tell you that when I read the paper I was very much astonished and delighted. I can say no more just now than to congratulate you warmly on the great discovery you have made and to renew my thanks to you for your kind- -ness in so early sending me your paper and the photographs.

Believe me,
Yours very truly,

Kelvin

Fig. 2.10 The congratulatory letter that Lord Kelvin wrote to Wilhelm Röntgen on 17 January 1896 following the discovery.

Reproduced with permission of the German Röntgen Museum.

Macintyre obtained the permission of the managers of Glasgow Royal Infirmary in March 1896 to set up an X-ray department, which was the first in the world. He was actively working on radiography and made the first demonstration of a renal stone, which was verified at surgery. The first issue of the journal *Archives of Clinical Skiagraphy* (the forerunner of the *British Journal of Radiology*) contained no less than three papers by Macintyre. He made his famous demonstration of the cineradiological study of the frog leg to the Royal Society of London in 1897 with a series of images to display the movement and reported his findings to Röntgen.

It was in 1897 that the famous electrical department opened at the Glasgow Royal Infirmary and rooms were fitted up with appropriate modern apparatus. What is quite remarkable is that wires were carried from the department to all the wards of the hospital to avoid the need to carry heavy apparatus. Electricity was supplied either by the 250V mains supply from Glasgow Corporation or from the department's own generator. Patients could either attend the department or could be examined in the wards or operating theatres, since these were all wired for electricity. The department provided both electrical (electrotherapeutic) and radiological services. The radiological services included plain film radiography, radiotherapy, foreign body localization, and stereoscopic radiography. What is always so very interesting is to see how very contemporary the concerns of Macintyre and the other pioneers were. In 1903 Macintyre stated that the new building from 1897 was being fully used and that the staff number had been increased to get through the large number of cases! The Electrical Pavilion had been built as large as possible in 1897 and by 1903 the demands upon it were far in excess of what could be accomplished. They had two medical officers, an unqualified assistant, and a staff of nurses. The role of the radiological nurse can be seen as crucial right back to the earliest days of radiology departments and is not a recent addition. By 1903 the Electrical Pavilion was taking 2000 radiographs each year and performing many fluoroscopic examinations. Macintyre felt that the most important introduction to the hospital was the electrotherapeutic department. In 1903 Macintyre was also looking forward to the rebuilding of the hospital and was hoping, as many generations of radiologists were to do in subsequent years, for still greater facilities. Macintyre was president of the Röntgen Society in 1900 to 1901 and he died on 29 October 1928 in his home city of Glasgow.

The early radiology departments arose from a variety of sources. Many hospitals already had electrotherapeutic or electrical departments and so acquiring X-ray apparatus was a straightforward progression, and such was the case at the Royal London Hospital and St Bartholomew's Hospital. Photography was well developed by the 1890s and was provided to the public by chemist shops (community pharmacists). Since these chemists were used to photography and the techniques needed, it was relatively easy for them to also acquire X-ray apparatus and provide a radiography service. Examples of this include the Royal Victoria Infirmary in Newcastle-upon-Tyne where local chemists were invited into the hospital to radiograph patients. Since many early departments originated in electrotherapy departments it was an obvious progression to practice radiotherapy. The early radiologists practised both diagnosis and therapy and it was not until the 1930s that the split into the professions of radiodiagnosis and radiotherapy was formalized in Britain; in continental Europe the two branches of radiology were to be closely linked for much longer.

Medico-legal radiology

Sir Arthur Schuster and the Nelson incident

It was at Nelson, a small Lancashire textile town, that the first diagnostic use of X-rays took place outside of a physics laboratory or hospital department for forensic purposes. Sir Arthur Schuster FRS was one of the first scientists to receive a copy of Röntgen's first communication and he was one of the first to point out the medical possibilities of X-rays and their practical significance.[13] Schuster had been born in 1851 in Frankfurt am Main in Germany and was a mathematical physicist. He was professor of physics at Owens College (now part of the University of Manchester) and he quickly saw the value of the discovery. On 23 April 1896 at 20 North Street in Nelson, Elizabeth Ann Hartley had been shot by her husband Hargreaves. Hargreaves Hartley was 27 years old and was apparently a jealous young man. He had accused his wife of infidelity and then on 23 April 1896 he shot her four times, the bullets entering her head and neck. The bullets injured her jaw, ear, and neck, and caused severe injuries. The medical practitioner in Nelson, a Dr W.G. Little, had worked at Owens College and therefore sent for Professor Schuster. Unfortunately Schuster was unwell and he therefore sent his two assistants to Nelson in his place. The delicate radiographic apparatus was taken to Nelson since the patient was too ill to be moved from her home. The first X-ray plate took an hour to complete and the second took about 70 minutes. The proceedings were observed by Dr Little, the mayor of Nelson, and the town clerk, and the plates were returned to Manchester for processing. Professor Schuster then telegrammed Dr Little saying that whilst the procedure had been successful there was some doubt about the location of the fourth bullet. When he had recovered from his illness Professor Schuster went to Nelson and took another radiograph. The final glass plate was probably placed underneath or behind Mrs Hartley's skull and Schuster was finally successful in locating the fourth bullet. Unfortunately, Mrs Hartley was too unwell to undergo surgery and she died on 9 May 1896. Professor Schuster subsequently gave a demonstration in the Lecture Room of the Technical School in Nelson of the radiographic techniques used. His subject for the demonstration was a Mrs Taylor of Boundary Street, Colne, who had a fragment of a broken needle retained in her hand for two years. The plate was developed by the photographer Mr J.L. Hopper of Pendle Street in Nelson. The exposure lasted about 5 minutes and the plate took around half an hour to develop. Whilst the Nelson incident is of interest, as Brogdon points out, since no treatment was possible and the patient died then this case 'can be considered an early manifestation of our tendency to use elaborate procedures and the newest technology, whether or not it will influence the outcome'.[14] However, the incident did illustrate the capabilities of the new technique and showed what would be possible in the future. Sir Arthur Schuster died in 1934 as one of the most famous professors in the Department of Physics and Astronomy at Manchester University.

Border control

That radiography could be used in areas other than the medical was obvious, including its use in customs and border control and this continues today. Fluoroscopy of suspect packages using the cryptoscope was being undertaken as early as 1897. The cryptoscope was a hooded fluorescent screen that could be brought to the eyes and which examined suspect packages placed in front of an X-ray tube. The technique was illustrated in the French periodical *L'Illustration* of 3 July 1897. The trade card illustrated was issued by Cacao Blooker. The front of the card illustrated a respectable woman with the name of the company as a series of apparently meaningless lines. The reverse of the card shows the cacao tin and more meaningless lines. When the card is transilluminated the name of the company is revealed and the contraband in the respectable lady's hand luggage is revealed. The apparatus that is now used for looking for items hidden under clothing and in luggage has reached a considerable degree of sophistication.

Postal security

There is now a considerable sophistication in examining the mail with radiography employed to look for letter bombs or illicit material sent through the postal service. In the UK many companies are on still on alert after a letter bomb campaign in early 2007 with explosives placed in party poppers in jiffy bags. Businesses need to have a mail security plan and maintain vigilance. Selected businesses may require special precautions with the use of a large-capacity cabinet postal X-ray scanner for checking letters, courier deliveries, parcels, and handbags.

X-ray surveillance

We now have available portable digital radiographic equipment, which can be used by police, military, customs, prisons, and building security managers for security checking unattended bags and suspicious packages. Other uses include bomb disposal, the search for narcotics and hidden contraband, searching behind walls for bugs/weapons, vehicle panel/tyre inspection, and non-destructive testing. In Chapter 4, Figure 4.4 shows an image from pre-1900 on a trade card of life as predicted in the year 2000 and is not so far from the truth. The policeman is looking through the wall to see the criminals robbing the safe. We can now obtain images of illicit goods and hidden items in trucks and vehicles and weapons concealed under clothes are revealed.

References

1. **Thomas, A.M.K.** (1995). Development of diagnostic radiology. In Thomas, A.M.K., Isherwood, I., and Wells, P.N.T (Eds), *The Invisible Light. 100 Years of Medical Radiology*, pp. 13–18. Oxford: Blackwell Science.

2. **Green, G.** (1999). *The Woman Who Knew Too Much: Alice Stewart and the Secrets of Radiation*. Ann Arbor, MI: The University of Michigan Press.

3. **Holland, C.T.** (1938). X-rays in 1896. *British Journal of Radiology*, *11*, 1–24.

4. **Holland, C.T.** (1895). *The Healing Art*. (Presidential address to the Liverpool Medico-Literary Society, 4 October.) Unpublished manuscript.

5. **Thomas, A.M.K.** (2010). Early forensic radiology. In Nushida, H., Vogel, H., Püschel, K., and Heinmann, A. (Eds), *Der durchsichtige Tote—Post mortem CT und forensische Radiologie*, pp. 103–115. Hamburg: Verlag Dr. Kovač.

6. **Dally, A.** (1996). *Fantasy Surgery 1880–1939*. Amsterdam: Rodopi.

7. **Köhler, A.** (1910). *Lexikon der Grenzen des Normalen und der Anfänge des Pathologischen im Röntgenbilde*. Hamburg: Lucas Gräfe & Sillem.

8. **Köhler, A.** (1931). *Röntgenology: The Borderlands of the Normal and Early Pathological in the Skiagram*. London: Ballière, Tindall & Cox.

9. **Köhler, A.** (1935). *Röntgenology: The Borderlands of the Normal and Early Pathological in the Skiagram* (2nd edn). London: Ballière, Tindall & Cox.

10. **Scott, S.G.** (1931). *Radiology in Relation to Medical Jurisprudence (Employer's Liability and Workmen's Compensation Acts)*. London: Cassell.

11. **Keats, K.E. and Anderson, M.W.** (2012). *Atlas of Normal Roentgen Variants That May Simulate Disease* (9th edn). Philadelphia, PA: Saunders.

12. **Clark, K.C.** (1939). *Positioning in Radiography*. London: Heinemann.

13. **Schuster, A.** (1932). *Reminiscences*. London: Macmillan.

14. **Brogdon, B.G. and Lichtenstein, J.E.** (1998). Forensic radiology in historical perspective. In Brogdon, B.G. (Ed.), *Forensic Radiology*, pp. 13–34. Boston, MA: CRC Press.

Chapter 3

Military radiology

As our technology has advanced, humans have developed increasingly sophisticated weapons for warfare and conflict, and as a result medicine has had to adapt to cope with the volume and the changing nature of resultant injuries. Following the discovery of X-rays in 1895 it became immediately apparent to military surgeons that this was a new technique that would be of great value in the treatment of war wounds.[1–4] The end of the 19th century was a period of rapidly changing military technology. As an example, the older and soft lead bullets were being replaced with new steel-jacketed bullets, and throughout the 1890s European governments were equipping their armies with new and more powerful magazine rifles, including the Martini–Henry and the Mauser. These new high-velocity bullets made a small entry wound and would often pass straight through the body. The older gaping entrance wounds were no longer seen and military surgeons realized that exploration of the wound for bullets was often more harmful for the patient than careful observation. The introduction of radiography allowed the military surgeon to locate any retained bullets. The younger generation of regimental surgeons who saw the value of X-rays was a generation trained in both the Listerian concepts of antisepsis and the germ theory of Louis Pasteur. In the UK many young doctors were attracted to the professional career provided by the newly established Royal Army Medical Corps, which set military medicine on to a professional footing. The technical aspects of radiography were not, however, easy and the early X-ray tubes were very fragile. However in spite of limitations, the apparatus available before 1900 could detect both fractures and foreign bodies.

The Royal Victoria Hospital was located at Netley near Southampton in England from 1856 until its final closure in 1978.[3] Military hospitals were increasing in importance and developments in artillery and infantry fire increased the proportion of the wounded as compared to those suffering from infectious diseases. In May 1896 there was a demonstration at Netley by Sidney Rowland (1872–1917) to Surgeon-Lieutenant-Colonel William F. Stevenson of a soldier with a complex tibial plateau fracture. Sidney Rowland was the editor of the *Archives of Clinical Skiagraphy*, which was the first radiological journal in the world and continues today as the *British Journal of Radiology*. The journalist William Dick observed, 'Of the scientific attainments brought to bear in treating the wounded here, I had an opportunity to form a judgement from personal observations. Colonel Stevenson and Major Dick, professors of surgery at the school, were engaged in experiments with the latest appliances for locating bullets by Röntgen rays...What bungling and haphazard all former methods seem to be by comparison with this!'[4] By mid-1898 X-ray sets were either being operated or were being installed at British military hospitals in Netley, Aldershot, Dublin, Woolwich (The Royal Herbert Hospital), and Gibraltar. Also of interest is that in 1903 the British Army Medical School at the Royal Victoria Hospital at Netley offered 'A course of X-ray instruction' and this was the origin of the first school of radiography in the world. In 1910 William F. Stevenson wrote that 'There is, of course, no question as to the necessity of x-ray apparatus and an officer qualified in its use being supplied to all general and stationary hospitals in war'.[5] All that is left now of the Royal Victoria Hospital is the chapel, which contains a museum.

The Italo-Abyssinian War

The first use of the X-rays in warfare was in the Italo-Abyssinian War of 1896 when the ancient kingdom of Abyssinia was invaded by Italian forces. The Italians lost at the battle at Adowa, which took place on 1 March 1896, and casualties were returned to the base hospitals in Italy by sea. Lieutenant-Colonel Giuseppe Alvaro was Medical Lieutenant Colonel and director of the Military Hospital at Naples and he gets the credit for taking the first radiographs of war casualties. He successfully took radiographs of two soldiers with fractures of their forearm bones using a Crookes tube and a Rühmkorff induction coil. It is remarkable that these radiographs were made only 6 months after the discovery of X-rays and they show clearly the presence of retained bullets. Colonel Alvaro stated that the new technique 'has proved to be a great aid in diagnosis, enabling us to determine with mathematical precision exactly where a foreign body was located'.[6]

The Greco-Turkish War

In the spring of 1897 fighting broke out in the Balkans and the various European powers were divided with Germany supporting the Turkish side and Britain, Russia, and the French supporting the Greeks. The German Red Cross Society immediately sent a unit to Constantinople and the *Daily Chronicle* (a London newspaper) sent two fully staffed and equipped modern hospital units to Greece under the British Red Cross with the surgeon Francis Abbott in charge. The British equipment included a complete modern X-ray apparatus similar to that in use at St Thomas's Hospital in London. Casualties were received from the Battle of Domoko, which took place on 17 May 1897. The X-ray apparatus was operated by Robert Fox Symons, and Francis Abbott gave an account of the various difficulties that were encountered. A room at the base hospital in Phalaerum was set out for the X-ray equipment and Fox Symons had this installed and working by 1 June 1897. Casualties arrived almost immediately and the X-ray work continued for about 6 weeks. There were many difficulties but, nevertheless, the overall results were very successful. It should be remembered that this was at a time when radiography was difficult, even in a modern hospital environment. Abbott and Fox Symons were able to illustrate their report about their activities with several radiographs and claimed 'to record the first skiagrams taken in wartime, as well as to show that even inexperienced hands working can get fair result'.[3] The original radiographic prints were exhibited in London at the first conversazione of the Röntgen Society (which became the British Institute of Radiology) that took place on 15 November 1897. Abbott and his team treated some 114 patients with war injuries and Fox Symons radiographed about half of them.

The account of Abbott and Fox Symons is interesting because it showed the use of X-rays under field conditions, and was the first time that radiography was used by the British Army and therefore influenced attitudes to subsequent campaigns. Fox Symons had hoped that it would be possible to use a fluorescent screen rather than simply taking radiographic plates, and therefore the retained bullet could be looked at in different projections and so this would avoid the need for the much slower process of obtaining a dry plate.

Fox Symons lists the technical difficulties, which included the heavy weight of the coil and accumulators, the fragility of the Crookes tubes and glass plates, the dangers of transporting cases of sulphuric acid for the accumulators, the delicacy and temperamental nature of the apparatus, and the general problems of transportation. An additional source of difficulty was the superstition of the local inhabitants who looked at the apparatus and its use as the work of the devil. Fox Symons said it was difficult to take radiographs when the patient was constantly making the sign of the cross over himself to ward off evil spirits! Probably the most serious obstacle to field radiography was the lack of reliable electrical power and this meant that the X-ray apparatus could not be located where it would be of most use, which was at Khalkis where the hospital nearest to the front line was located. Even Phalaerum did not have access to a mains electrical supply and so the Royal Navy warship HMS *Rodney* was used as the source of electricity to allow them to recharge their wet batteries.

The casualties consisted mainly of possible fractures or suspected retained bullets with several patients having wounds with bullets penetrating body cavities. The results of radiography not only helped with the immediate treatment of the patient but also defined a new area of military medicine. As has been said, the nature of war wounds was changing due to the newer high-velocity rifles and Abbott wrote to the War Office saying that:

> The Roentgen rays should always, if possible, be available at the hospital nearest the front in which the wounds can be first properly examined and dealt with…the apparatus is of no use in the field where detection can only be an incentive to premature exploration. The less wounds are tampered with before satisfactory surroundings are reached, the better. The modern bullet…is practically aseptic and there is no urgency for removal.[6]

Walter Caverley Beevor and the Tirah Campaign

In June 1897 there was an insurrection in the Northwest frontier of India on the frontier with Afghanistan and a British Army was sent to open up the mountain passes. The Tirah Expeditionary Force consisted of 8000 British and 30,000 Indian soldiers under the command of General Sir William Lockhart. A total of 23 field hospitals were established on the Tirah Plateau and 900 casualties were received. The geography necessitated a long journey back to the base hospital at Rawalpindi with very slow transport of the wounded, and as a result the military surgeons treated wounds earlier and nearer to the front line than would be usual.

Walter Caverley Beevor (1858–1927) was a Regimental Surgeon with the Coldstream Guards and he used X-rays to examine 200 patients on the Tirah Plateau, later taking further X-rays in the hospital at Rawalpindi. Beevor had been attached to the Brigade of Guards and had obtained permission to go out to India for a year. He had brought with him his Röntgen X-ray apparatus that he had purchased at his own expense from the firm A.E. Dean in Hatton Gardens in London. Beevor joined a field hospital and was able to use his apparatus. He had purchased three X-ray tubes and was able to show the position of bullets that could not otherwise be found. The X-rays were also thought excellent when negative results were found and the presence of a retained bullet was excluded. The examinations included the leg of General Woodhouse himself, whose leg wound had failed to heal satisfactorily, and some weeks following the injury Beevor was able to show a retained bullet. That Walter Beevor could take his primitive apparatus to such a remote location is quite remarkable and a testament to his skills.

Beevor made a presentation to the United Services Institution in May 1898 when he returned to England. It was concluded that radiography alleviated the sufferings of many wounded men and the preservation of limbs and that a Röntgen ray apparatus 'would seem to be a very great addition to the medical equipment of a force'.[7] This view was soon implemented and Beevor's work marked the introduction of field radiography units to the British Army.

John Battersby and the River War

In 1898 a British army of 20,000 men equipped with modern weapons and led by General Herbert Kitchener was sent from Cairo to the Sudan against the Mahdists. The force was taken up the Nile by Thomas Cook's pleasure boats as far as the cataract at Aswan. In the battle at Omdurman on 1 September in broad daylight, 50,000 Mahdist tribesmen armed with only spears and primitive guns attacked this modern army and the casualties were frightful. The slaughter led Hilaire Belloc to write, 'Whatever happens, we have got the Maxim Gun and they have not'.[8]

The Army Medical Department had learnt from the experience of Walter Beevor and had ordered a portable apparatus from A.E. Dean to accompany the expedition but the X-ray apparatus was only sent after angry words in the British Parliament. The preliminary battle at Berber had already been fought when a Member of Parliament asked about the supply of X-ray apparatus. The Financial Secretary of the War Office then reported that the senior medical officer had stated that no patient would have been helped if radiography had not been available. A decision was finally made to send X-ray apparatus, and it was put in charge of Surgeon-Major John Battersby.

Battersby examined about 60 casualties at Abadieh near Berber on the upper Nile between July and October of 1898. Battersby's mud hut at Abadieh thereby became a landmark in the history of radiology and of military medicine because the apparatus that he used was provided by the War Office as part of regular medical supplies and was not the private property of the Medical Officer.

Battersby's main difficulties were related to the climate in the Sudan, and it was with great difficulty that the apparatus was made to work. The electricity was generated by a soldier using a stationary bicycle equipped with a dynamo. After the battle of Omdurman 121 wounded were sent for surgical treatment and in 21 patients conventional treatment could not find a bullet. In 20 of these patients an accurate diagnosis could be made using radiography and suffering was prevented by unnecessary probing of the wound. The 21st case was of a soldier who was too sick to be examined. Afterwards a senior surgeon commented that the X-rays had been of inestimable value by either avoiding unnecessary exploration or by accurately locating the position of the bullet. When Battersby returned to the UK he presented his findings to the Röntgen Society in January 1899. In addition to simple radiography Battersby used the famous cross-thread localization device developed by James Mackenzie Davidson to locate foreign bodies.

The Spanish–American War

Radiography was used in the Spanish–American War of 1898 and again unnecessary probing of the wound was avoided.[7] The larger American general hospitals and three hospital ships were all supplied with radiographic apparatus. The official view of the American forces was that the use of radiography in the field was unnecessary because the bullet wounds rarely required immediate removal and it was also believed that, since aseptic surgery was not easy under field conditions, if a radiograph could be obtained it would only encourage the surgeons to operate inappropriately. Captain William Borden published his document on the use of X-rays with an extensive account of the use of the new technique. The new technique was not without hazards and two cases of X-ray burns caused by repeated and prolonged exposure were presented. Borden believed that the most important factors responsible for the radiation burns were the duration of X-ray exposure and the closeness of the X-ray tube to the patient.

The Boer War

In 1899 hostilities started in South Africa. The initial preparations for the conflict were inadequate on the British side and what was expected to be only a brief conflict turned into a full-scale war. The British public had been told the fighting would be over by Christmas 1899 but the reality was that the fighting was to last fully two and a half years. The Boer War was the first occasion since the Crimea that the British Army faced an opponent with modern weapons. There were 500,000 British troops in South Africa of whom fewer than 6000 died in battle and more than 16,000 died of disease. The Boers lost the conflict with about 5000 dead.[3]

The medical arrangements became more sophisticated as the war progressed with a system of general (fixed) hospitals and field (moveable) hospitals. While the X-ray apparatus was supplied to the general hospitals as part of their essential equipment for the campaign, both electrical and radiation protection were still primitive. The general hospitals (but not the field hospitals) had portable X-ray apparatus to allow retained bullets to be detected and fractures to be diagnosed and treated. The equipment was now also supplied with a dynamo fitted with a motorcycle engine to generate the power needed for the batteries.

The apparatus provided consisted of:

- A 10-inch induction coil (Apps Newton), with condenser, spring-hammer interrupter, rods, and electrical cables, all packed in a teak case.
- Two six-cell lithanode accumulators.
- Six focus tubes (Cox's 'Record') with tube stand, each packed separately in a box.
- Mackenzie Davidson's cross-thread localizer with stand in a teak box.
- Nine dozen photographic glass plates (Edwards' cathodal plates), photographic paper, and chemicals.
- A 2½ horsepower motorcycle engine and dynamo.

Figure 3.1, entitled 'Science to the rescue. Finding a bullet with the X-ray apparatus at the military hospital, Pietermaritzburg', is taken from the *Black and White Budget* of 1899. The dramatic image with the X-ray tube looking like a light bulb in the centre above the patient shows the complete absence of both electrical and radiation protection that was characteristic of that time. However, of more immediate concern is the position of the left hand of the central figure who seems to be reaching out to touch the high-tension cables! Touching the exposed cables would result in death or a severe electric shock. Whilst this technology looks unbelievably primitive to us now, it should be remembered that at the time it was cutting-edge technology being utilized in difficult conditions. It was the experience of the Boer War that finally established radiology as an essential feature of modern military surgery.

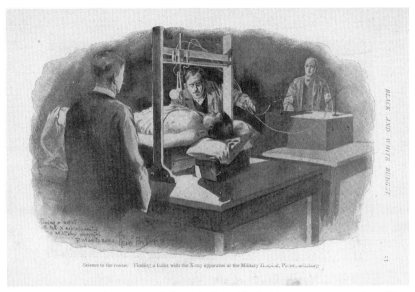

Fig. 3.1 'Science to the rescue. Finding a bullet with the X-ray apparatus at the military hospital, Pietermaritzburg.' *Black and White Budget*, 1899.

Reproduced from *Black and White Budget*, Black and White Publishing Co Ltd, UK, Copyright © 1899. Image courtesy of Dr Adrian M.K. Thomas.

Marie Curie and the First World War

The First World War with its tragic consequences resulted in a large number of casualties and put a considerable strain on casualty clearing and the mobile field hospitals. At the start of the war radiographic equipment was located in the larger army hospitals behind the front line. Initially it was believed there was no need for radiography to be available close to the fighting but as the war progressed the confidence of the army surgeons in the value of rapid radiography increased and this was a view also held by Marie Curie.[9] In France, Marie Curie developed an X-ray car (voiture radiologique) and she equipped 18 such cars herself (Figure 3.2). The motors of these cars could supply the current supply for the X-ray apparatus. Marie Curie also established 200 fixed radiographic units. As the war continued, the need for both radiologists and technicians increased. For example, the French radiologist Antoine Béclère developed a training school at Val-de-Grace Hospital and

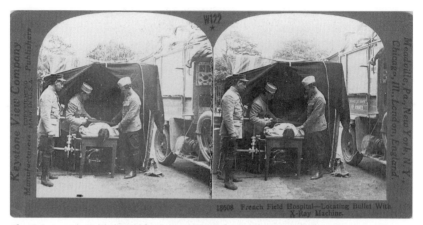

Fig. 3.2 French Field Hospital—locating bullet with X-ray machine (stereoscopic photographs).

Image produced by Keystone View Company, USA, circa 1910. Image courtesy of Dr Adrian M.K. Thomas.

the French Army opened a school for X-ray technicians. Marie Curie (Figure 3.3) opened a school for female X-ray technicians (manipulatrices) in 1916 and worked there with her daughter Irène.

At the beginning of hostilities, the European armies were supplied with the traditional gas (or ion) X-ray tubes. However, technology was developing and more powerful radiographic apparatus became available as the Coolidge tube and the Potter–Bucky diaphragm were introduced into radiological practice. The American Expeditionary force was supplied with the best radiographic apparatus available and these modern advances were utilized fully.

Following injury, the casualty was sent to a regimental aid post and then by a field ambulance to a casualty clearing station located some miles behind the front. If radiography were required then the patient would be transferred to the radiographic room. Most of the radiographic work consisted in the detection of retained bullets and only simple apparatus was needed. The stretcher with the patient was placed on supports above a moveable X-ray tube. The patient was rapidly fluoroscoped, and, using a parallax technique with tube movement (an early variant of tomography), the depth of the foreign body and its relation to the point of entry could be determined quickly and a written report

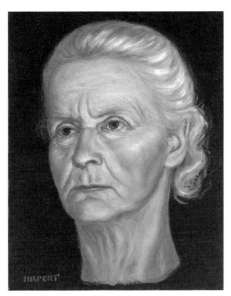

Fig. 3.3 Marie Curie. Painting by Josef Hilpert.
Image courtesy of Dr Adrian M.K. Thomas.

issued. The apparatus was also powerful enough to diagnose thoracic injuries and the use of stereoscopy was common.

The drawing in Figure 3.4 is from *Our Hospital ABC* which was published in the Great War and illustrated by Joyce Dennys. The 'ABC' stands for Anzac British Canadian and the book celebrated military hospitals. There was an illustration for each letter and the illustration for X is for 'The X-Ray' and notes 'If by any ill luck you swallow a sixpence it shows where it's stuck'. The apparatus illustrated looks like the radiographic apparatus in the old Ontario Military Hospital in south London, a 2000-bed hospital that became Orpington Hospital. These were the days before image intensification and radiography was commonly used to locate more serious foreign bodies than the old 6d coin (2½p)!

Vincent Cirillo has commented on the importance of the First World War for the general development of the speciality of radiology.[10] The army surgeons became accustomed to working in a team with radiologists and this practice continued in civilian clinical practice after the war.

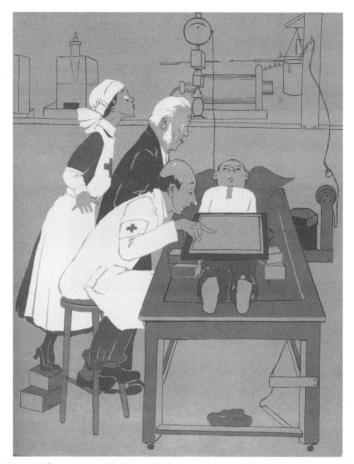

Fig. 3.4 Army fluoroscopy, The letter 'X from *Our Hospital ABC*. 'The X-Ray. If by any luck you swallow a sixpence it shows where it's stuck'.

Reproduced from *Our Hospital ABC* by Hampden Gordon and M. C. Tindall. Published by Bodley Head. Reprinted by permission of The Random House Group Limited.

The number of radiologists increased following the First World War and the X-ray equipment became easier to use; there was no lingering doubt that this war finally legitimized the discipline of military radiology.

Florence Stoney

Florence Ada Stoney (1870–1932)[11] (Figure 3.5) was born and grew up in Dublin, in Ireland, which was then part of the UK. She was educated at home and at the Royal College of Science. In the Cambridge

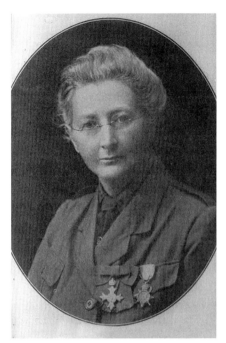

Fig. 3.5 Dr Florence Stoney, the pioneer female radiologist.

Reproduced with permission from *British Journal of Radiology*, Vol. *5*, No. 59, pp. 853–858, Copyright © 1932 British Institute of Radiology, DOI: 10.1259/0007-1285-5-59-853. Image kindly supplied by the archive of the British Institute of Radiology.

Higher Local examination she took First Class Honours in Natural Science and First Class Honours in Mathematics. Her father was Dr Johnstone Stoney FRS who supported the higher education of women and was involved in the founding of Girton College, Cambridge. At that time she could not study medicine at Dublin University since women were not admitted to medical degrees in Ireland and so she came to England, attending the London School of Medicine for Women and the Royal Free Hospital, graduating MB BS in 1895 with honours. She received the prize for the best student in her year and she obtained her MD in 1898. The London School of Medicine for Women was founded in 1874 by Miss Sophia Jex-Blake and linked to the Royal Free Hospital in 1877. The female medical pioneer Dr Elizabeth Garrett Anderson (1836–1917) was the Dean from 1883–1903 when Florence was a student at the school. Elizabeth Garrett Anderson was the first woman in

Britain to obtain a legal qualification as physician and surgeon and was the first woman dean of a medical school. Her example would have been inspiring to the young Florence Stoney.

For 6 years Florence was demonstrator in anatomy at the London School of Medicine for Women and this only stopped when it became apparent that there was no possibility of a woman being appointed to a lectureship.

In 1902 Florence Stoney started the X-ray departments at both the Royal Free Hospital and the New Hospital for Women (The Elizabeth Garrett Anderson Hospital) in London. She set up the X-ray departments at a time when the apparatus was still very primitive. The rooms were badly ventilated with no separate room for X-ray work. The X-ray department was initially left open for all to use but it had to be locked after the equipment was damaged. She often took the photographic plates home and developed them in her bathroom in the evenings. She had no assistant and she had to do all the work herself. At that time the radiologist was not even a member of the hospital medical staff and she was not a member of the committee that discussed the work of the X-ray department. The work that she undertook was varied and included examinations for foreign bodies (soft tissue and oesophageal), bullet wounds and fractures, examination for phthisis (tuberculosis) both pulmonary and articular, coxa vara, pes cavus, and treatments including rodent ulcer.

Unfortunately in 1907 the Royal Free Hospital appointed a man, Dr Harrison Orton, to take charge of the combined Department of Radiology and Electrotherapy and the appointment was made over her head. Florence Stoney continued with her X-ray work including treatment with X-rays of exophthalmic goitre (Grave's disease). Dr Orton resigned in 1913 and Florence Stoney left the Royal Free Hospital at the start of the First World War.

Florence Stoney visited the USA just before the outbreak of the First World War to see the X-ray work and gave a most interesting account in the *Archives of the Roentgen Ray* (the forerunner of the *British Journal of Radiology*) in October 1914. She visited the eastern USA towns and also Schenectady. She found the doctors very helpful and commented,

'I found the doctors in America, both in the hospitals and in private, very ready to allow me to see the work in their departments—medical women not being kept out of everything so much as in England'.[11] In America she found there was a major concern for radiation protection. For example, nowhere was the operator left exposed to radiation apart for fluoroscopy and there was only a limited use of fluoroscopy. She described the use of a mirror to observe the fluorescent screen with the operator being protected behind a lead screen. Bismuth (not barium at that time) was used for gastrointestinal diagnosis and from six to 40 radiographs were taken to diagnose gastric and duodenal ulcers in those days before modern endoscopy. It was common practice to include a reduced-sized print of the abnormality with the written report. The newly invented Coolidge X-ray tube was seen in frequent use. The Coolidge tube is the modern type of tube with a hot spiral cathode and high vacuum that replaced the older cold cathode gas tubes. Significantly she brought back a new Coolidge X-ray tube which was only the second to arrive in England.

Florence Stoney also saw treatment with irradiation during her visit to the USA. This was mainly carried out using radium emanation that was contained in small metal needles that inserted directly into the tumour. She visited Philadelphia and observed radiotherapy with X-rays. She was impressed by the treatment of a 36-year-old woman with breast cancer who was treated directly after surgery. She said they used heavy doses, heavily filtered and frequently repeated. The surface was carefully marked out and exposed in turn with a crossfire being directed on the tumour from as many points as possible.

In the spring of 1914 Florence and her sister Edith had a complete portable X-ray installation prepared including the Coolidge tube that she had acquired in the USA. This apparatus had been put together by the sisters to give medical assistance in the event of a possible civil war in Ireland. On 4 August 1914, the first day of the First World War, Florence and Edith Stoney were able to offer their services to the British Red Cross at the War Office in London. By this time, she had 13 years' experience in radiology and was very experienced. Her offer was refused by Sir Frederick Treves because she was a woman. It was said that she 'wasted no time with arguments or indignation' and cooperated with the author Mrs St. Clair Stobart in organizing a voluntary women's unit. This unit was established with the Belgian Red Cross and consisted of 100 (later 135) beds, six women doctors, ten trained nurses, and female orderlies. Florence organized the medical part of the surgical unit that was staffed entirely by women and was the Principal Medical Officer and Radiologist. Initially they went to Brussels and were turned back. However, in September 1914 they went to Antwerp and set up their all-woman's hospital described as 'a model of organization'.

The Stobart Hospital in Antwerp had 100 beds located in an old concert hall, and it was established before the 'official' British Army hospitals had been set up. Florence wrote to Edith about the progress on 23 September 1914. The unit saw many casualties straight from the trenches. On 8 October 1914 they were under shellfire for 18 hours and their situation became desperate. They evacuated their patients and then started to walk to Holland and were picked up by three London buses and had to sit on ammunition cases. The use of mechanical transport in warfare on a large scale for the first time enabled the rapid concentration of troops at any given point and was a major reason why large numbers of casualties were possible. The buses were used to transport troops and ammunition from the railhead to the back of the firing line. The road out of Antwerp was described by Florence as a sad procession of fleeing peasants, troops, cattle, guns, wagons, children, and carts, all moving in the same direction as rapidly as possible. She escaped from Antwerp only 20 minutes before the bridge was blown up. She continued work in France and re-established a hospital near Cherbourg. Florence was 'Radiographer and Head of the Staff' at this Anglo-French Hospital, No 2, Chateau Tourlaville, Cherbourg which was under the care of the British Red Cross and St John's Ambulance. The disused chateau was transformed into a modern hospital. Water, sanitation, and electricity had to be arranged and the X-ray equipment was again primitive and many difficulties were encountered. Their patients were seriously wounded, many with septic fractures. The radiographs were used to show the positions of the fractures and location of the shrapnel and bullet which could then be extracted. The X-ray apparatus had been given privately and she made use of her Coolidge tube. Full use was made of localizing devices for foreign bodies including the Mackenzie Davidson localizing stand and the Pirie stereoscope. The surgeons required as much help as possible to locate and remove small pieces of broken rifle bullets.

Florence wrote:

> We horrified the French by insisting on fresh air, with the result that all visitors, medical as well as lay, remarked how ruddy and well our patients looked, unlike the white faces you see in most of the hospitals. The Consulting Surgeon for the whole of the Cherbourg district came to see our hospital, thinking it was a waste of time to go to a place only staffed by women doctors, but after spending a couple of hours going thoroughly round the wards he wrote 'L'hôpital de Tourlaville est très bien organisé, les malades sont très bien soignés, et les chirurgiennes sont de valeur égale aux chirurgiens les meilleurs' ['The hospital of Tourlaville is very well organized, the sick are very well treated, and the surgeons are of a value equal to the best'].[11]

The patients were also appreciative and Lance-Corporal F. Reynolds of the 2nd Oxford and Bucks Light Infantry wrote in the *Daily News* of 9 January 1915, 'Lady doctors do all the work—no men at all, so you can guess I am all right. George and I were the only two spared out of six in our trench. Don't you think I had a fine birthday?'.[12]

Attitudes gradually changed, partly because of practical necessity, and in March 1915 Florence was one of five women doctors accepted for full-time work under the War Office by Sir Alfred Keogh. She was appointed as Head of the 'X-ray and Electrical Department' of the Fulham Military Hospital and when she took up her post was the first woman doctor to work under the War Office in England. The hospital had more than 1000 beds and she personally examined more than 15,000 cases. Her work was concerned particularly with the localization of bullets and her knowledge of anatomy helped the surgeons greatly. She also was able to identify the presence of sequestra (dead bone) and the removal of this aided the treatment of these injuries significantly. She developed an interest in soldier's heart and in shell shock and believed that some cases were related to hyperthyroidism. For her war work she was awarded the OBE in 1919. For her services she was also decorated and the 1914 Star with bar as given for service under fire, the British

War Medal, the Victory Medal with oak leaf for mention in despatches, and the British Red Cross Medal. She was also awarded the newly set up radiological examination diploma, the Cambridge DMRE, honoris causa in 1920 because of her past experience.

Her health was damaged by the war, related in part to her overexposure to radiation, and she was observed to have X-ray dermatitis of her left hand. Florence moved to Bournemouth on the south coast of England where she was on the staff of two hospitals. She was Honorary Medical Officer to the Electrical Department of the Royal Victoria and West Hants Hospital in Bournemouth and was the founder and president of the Wessex branch of the British Institute of Radiology. She retired from her hospital appointments in 1928. During her career she was concerned with women's health issues including the treatment of fibroids and the diagnosis of pelvic deformities in women due to osteomalacia that would cause problems in childbirth. In retirement she travelled in India to investigate osteomalacia and this was the subject of her last scientific paper. Florence Stoney died in 1932 at the age of 62. She had a 'gentle kindness and rich sympathy for suffering—showed courage in her own last, long and painful illness'.[11] Her obituary in the *British Journal of Radiology* covered five pages and contained many warm personal testimonials.

Florence Stoney had a firm faith in the potential capacity of women to fill positions of the highest responsibility. She felt that women should develop their powers to the highest possible extent and then, if opportunity failed them, they should make their own opportunity. She was a keen constitutional Suffragist (Suffragette) pressing for votes for women and she took part in many demonstrations and processions. In personality she was shy and retiring with a quiet manner. This was combined with an iron will and undaunted courage. Her gentle graciousness disarmed opposition and gained cooperation: 'few had dreamt of the ardour existing beneath that demure and gentle exterior'.[11] In professional matters she was very keen to pass on all that she learnt. She was innovative in her approach to radiology and was involved in many early X-ray developments. Her life remains an inspiration.

The Second World War

By 1939 good, reliable, shockproof portable apparatus was available and radiological services were generally well organized. The British Army was supplied with a good mobile X-ray machine, the MX2, which was robust and easy to use for both radiography and fluoroscopy. It could easily be put into a crate for transportation but packing the apparatus was not always easy. By this period radiography had developed as a profession and many radiographers entered the forces; however, overall numbers of radiologists and radiographers available were inadequate and many units were supplied with radiographers only, without medical radiologists. The numbers of radiographers meant that on average 50 to 100 patients could be dealt with each day and the War Office recommended that if this number were exceeded then the lightly wounded and the prisoners of war should be asked to help the radiographer. There were no radiologists in the casualty clearing stations or in the forward area and the full responsibility for the work rested with the radiographer. These radiographers developed considerable skills and were integral to the team, and professional skills were more important than the exact military rank. The radiation dangers of fluoroscopy were well realized and it was not recommended unless performed under expert supervision.

In the US forces, two radiologists were assigned to each mobile surgical hospital unit. The work would consist of fluoroscopy of casualties, foreign body localization, and general duties. There was also radiotherapy for superficial infections including gas gangrene in this time before the introduction of antibiotics. Compared to the First World War, the action was more mobile and radiographic units accompanied the field hospitals.

Post 1945

There were no significant changes to radiological technology during the Korean War (1950–1953). During the Vietnam War (1965–1973) American military hospitals were equipped with high-powered apparatus. It was possible to rapidly transfer patients from the battlefield to the hospital with a helicopter transit to the MASH (Mobile Army Surgical Hospital) with an average time of 15 minutes. There was a significant use of civilian hospitals and since this equipment was an old legacy of the French colonial rule it was quite primitive. For example, barium gastrointestinal studies had to be performed using plain films since fluoroscopy was seldom available. Radiography at the field hospitals was essential since it enabled the surgeons to decide who could be treated locally and who needed to be transferred to the base hospital.

Technology continues to develop and since the early 1980s there are available special expandable radiological containers fitted with radiographic fluoroscopic equipment. As civilian technology has developed, so the knowledge has been applied to military medicine. One significant innovation is teleradiology, the remote viewing of radiological images. As an example, in Bosnia in 2002 it was possible for the digital radiographic images of a US soldier to be transmitted using teleradiology links, first to the Landstuhl Regional Medical Center in Germany and from there to the Walter Reed Army Medical Center in Washington, DC, in the USA. This new development has solved one of the long-standing problems for military doctors, namely the absence of specialist medical advice and the dangers of professional isolation. The US military developed a 'Deployable Radiology' (DepRad) system, a teleradiology network designed by Georgetown University, Washington, DC. The service was also used to provide a service for Camp Doha-Kuwait where there were no radiologists on site. One of the problems with military radiology is that there are not enough radiologists to cover every unit. For example, in the Second World War many surgical units had no radiologist and the radiographer was often called upon to provide the diagnosis. The DepRad was designed to provide a global radiology service both for US soldiers and for their families. The US military authorities have been extremely forward thinking in implementing modern digital technology and military hospitals are being supplied with computed radiography and picture archiving and communication systems (PACS) that can even support forward deployed combat support hospitals.

Teleradiology can also help the continuing problem of inadequate and falling numbers of military radiologists. The military staffing issues mirror civilian ones with increasing workloads in radiology departments and the difficulties of supporting the new radiological modalities and the large numbers of images. In February 2003 more than 1350 radiological studies comprising 15,300 images were transmitted over the Landstuhl's teleradiology network.[13] Once the radiological images are available on PACS the radiological reporting can be outsourced to a civilian radiology practice, although as with all transmission of medical images, secure and encrypted links are vital on account of the significant security issues.

In more recent years modern digital radiology systems have become available. These systems are lightweight, robust, and portable, and the digital image is transferred without the need for film processing. The processing of radiological films in the field has always been difficult whether it has been in a tent on the banks of the Nile in 1898 or in a field hospital in Vietnam in 1966. However, digital technology need not be complex and clinical images have been recorded on a mobile telephone and sent as a text message!

Nevertheless, reliance on digital technology may prove problematic. In addition to conventional warfare there is now an emerging 'Web War' with attacks that result in a 'denial of service'. In October 2010 the UK government announced that £650 million would be allocated to combating cyber warfare and the threat is very real. What has been called Web War 1 was launched against Estonia in 2007, and Russia mounted a cyber-attack before its conventional invasion of Georgia in 2008.[14]

The military surgeons at the end of the 19th century rapidly realized the value of radiography in military surgery and innumerable lives and limbs have been saved as a result. As military technology developed, so did the technology to treat war casualties. We owe a debt to the early pioneers who initiated the development of military radiology, the need for which is sadly still very much with us.

References

1. **Guy, J.M.** (1995). British military radiology, 1897–1919. In Thomas, A.M.K., Isherwood, I., and Wells, P.N.T. (Ed.), *The Invisible Light. 100 Years of Medical Radiology*, pp. 39–41. Oxford: Blackwell Science.

2. **Reynolds, L.** (1945). The history of the use of the roentgen ray in warfare. *American Journal of Roentgenology*, *54*, 649–672.

3. **Burrows, E.H.** (1986). *Pioneers and Early Years: A History of British Radiology*. Alderney: Colophon.

4. **Hoare, P.** (2001). *Spike Island: A Memoir of a Military Hospital*. London: Fourth Estate.

5. **Stevenson, W.F.** (1910). *Wounds in War: The Mechanism of their Production and Treatment*. London: Longmans Green.

6. **Thomas, A.M.K.** (2000). The first 50 years of military radiology 1895–1945. *European Journal of Radiology*, *63*, 214–219.

7. **Shadwell, L.J.** (1898). *Lockhart's Advance through Tirah*. London: W. Thacker.

8. **Keown-Boyd, H.** (1986). *A Good Dusting: A Centenary Review of the Sudan Campaigns 1883–1899*. London: Guild Publishing.

9. **Quinn, S.** (1995). *Marie Curie: A Life*. London: Heinemann.

10. **Cirillo, V.J.** (2000). The Spanish–American War and military radiology. *American Journal of Roentgenology*, *174*, 1233–1239.

11. **Thomas, A.M.K.** (2010). Florence Stoney and early British military radiology. In Nushida, H., Vogel, H., Püschel, K., and Heinmann, A. (Eds), *Der durchsichtige Tote—Post mortem CT und forensische Radiologie*, pp. 103–113. Hamburg: Verlag Dr. Kovač.

12. (1915). *Daily News*, 9 January.

13. **Page, D.** Teleradiology is the new Army medical mule. [Online.] Available at: <http://home.earthlink.net/~douglaspage/id62.html>.

14. **Coghlan, T. and Haynes, D.** (2011). WWII. *The Times (Eureka)*, *19*, 38–42.

Chapter 4

Radiology and popular culture

There is a long-standing interaction between science and popular culture and many medical images and themes in literature, advertising, and films.

Radiology and paper ephemera

In recent years there has been an increasing interest in printed ephemera.[1] The term ephemera covers a wide variety of printed material. The word ephemera comes from the Greek and refers to the flies that only live for a day. Maurice Rickards, the founder of Ephemera Society in the UK, has defined ephemera as 'the minor transient documents of everyday life'.[2] This definition is not altogether satisfactory because while the papers may be for transient use, at the time they may be significant and considerable effort may have been put into their design and printing. John Johnson made the collection of ephemera that is now at the Bodleian Library in Oxford and he was one of the first 20th-century scholars to recognize the importance of paper ephemera. There are several collections of medical paper ephemera including those at the Wellcome Library in London and the Thackray Museum in Leeds, and a Centre for Ephemera Studies based in the University of Reading, UK.

Radiological ephemera

Ephemera in radiology may be divided into material that that has been produced by radiology departments, by the X-ray industry, and the purely popular.[3,4] The material arising from the radiology departments is of great interest and provides significant information on how radiology departments have worked throughout the years. This material consists of request forms, radiological reports, letters, and patient information material. Unfortunately, there has been no systematic collection of these items and indeed there is no systematic collection of X-ray films and plates showing the examinations that have been performed during the history of radiology.

Trade cards

Trade cards originated as the printed cards that were given away by shopkeepers and traders to advertise their services.[5] The production of trade cards was stimulated by the development of the technique of chromolithography in the mid-19th century. The process of chromo-lithography was complex with a series of colours added sequentially to produce a high-quality multicolour image. The cards produced were called 'chromos' and they were collected keenly. This collection would encourage loyalty to the shop or product. The first use was at the shop A Bon Marché in Paris. The proprietor was Jacques-Aristide Boucicaut who initially was a partner but who took over the business in 1863. The shop developed from a small shop to the largest dry goods business in the world. Over 400 sets of cards were issued by the firm, often in sets of six or more. The cards could be pasted into an album. This idea was soon copied and many businesses produced the new cards. These attractive cards were made at a time when the possibility of having quality colour illustrations in magazines and newspapers was limited and the cards were instantly popular and heavily collected.

The Suchard card shown in Figure 4.1 has an illustration of Wilhelm Röntgen and early radiology apparatus. The X-ray tube is a simple glass bulb and examples of radiographs are shown on the walls of the room. The image is an evocative memory of the early days of radiology. Philippe Suchard (1797–1884) opened his first confectionary shop in Neuchatel in Switzerland in 1825. Suchard pioneered the building of houses for his workers and in 1846 he established an Alpine village for Swiss immigrants to the USA. In 1859, with Henri Dunant the founder of the Red Cross, he helped the wounded after the battle of Solferino. Suchard started issuing trade cards in 1880–1883 and they proved immensely popular and are actively collected today. The idea was soon copied. Printing firms pre-pared stock designs and so the same image could be used by more than one company. Many firms produced these cards including manufacturers

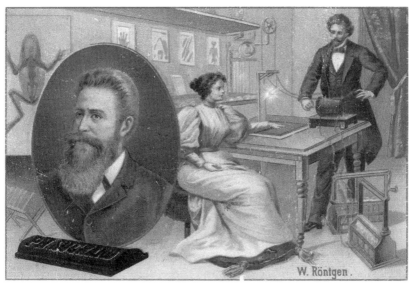

Fig. 4.1 Wilhelm Röntgen depicted on a Suchard trade card, c.1900.

Card published by Suchard Chocolate, Switzerland, c.1900. Image courtesy of Dr Adrian M.K. Thomas.

of coffee, tea, malted drinks, and confectionary including Suchard. Of particular interest is the firm of Guérin-Boutron of Paris, who produced numerous cards with a radiological theme.

Cigarette and tobacco cards

Cigarette cards originated as a stiffening card inserted into packets of cigarettes.[5] They were first produced in America in the late 1870s. The early topics for the cards were of glamour, military, and sporting themes since the first smokers were almost exclusively men. As the popularity of the cards and cigarettes increased so did the topics on the cards. Large series of cards were issued and the craze for collecting reached its peak in the first period of the 20th century up to about 1940. Radiographic topics are quite common on tobacco cards and include Wilhelm Röntgen, the X-ray tube, and radiotherapy.

Picture postcards

The modern postcard was introduced in the Austro-Hungarian Empire in October 1869 and was introduced in the UK on 1 October 1870.[6]

Dr Emanuel Herman wrote an article entitled Uber eine neue Art der Korrespondenz mittels der Post (A new way of correspondence by post) which appeared in the *Neue Freie Presse* on 26 January 1869 encouraging the use of a postal card. The early postal cards were made of a buff card and measured 89×122mm. In the United Kingdom the postage rate for these new cards was only ½d as opposed to the ordinary rate of 1d. The commercial benefit was soon realized and these postcards became immensely popular, particularly in the period leading up to the First World War with many millions of cards being printed. The style of writing on these new cards was different from the older verbose letters and the texts on the cards had to be brief. A new form of communication developed in much the same way that modern e-mail and text messages are changing the way we communicate today. Pictures were soon printed on the cards and there were many themes. These themes could be comical, propaganda, advertising, novelty, and miscellaneous. The novelty card shown in Figure 4.2 is interesting. In the centre of the star is a grid. When the fingers are looked at through the grid the penumbra gives the illusion of seeing the bones and is the basis of the X-ray spectacles (X-ray Spex) popular in the 1950s. Postcard collecting is a very popular hobby today with many fairs still being held each weekend.

Miscellaneous material

The penguin on the wrapper for a Penguin chocolate bar shown in Figure 4.3 is using the X-ray machine to view the fish he has just eaten. Although the wrapper is recent, the apparatus used is of 1930s vintage. This wrapper is classic ephemera. The term ephemera does not imply that the object is of poor quality. The wrapper is well designed and produced and considerable thought must have been given to the design of the picture. However, the wrapper is transient and once used is thrown away.

Themes in popular radiological ephemera

The first and most enduring theme is the reality that we are all walking skeletons. The X-rays remind us of this unpleasant but obvious truth.

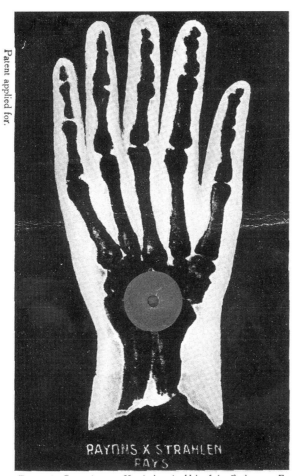

To see the Bones in your Hand place the Hole of the Card to your Eye. and your Hand, with fingers apart, 12 inches distant in front of a window.

Fig. 4.2 X-ray post card giving the illusion of X-ray vision when the hand is viewed through the gridded aperture.

Published by Nels, Brussels, c.1900. Image courtesy of Dr Adrian M.K. Thomas.

This theme is found in the earliest years of radiography and is disturbing to our normal view of ourselves. The X-rays reveal something that should be kept hidden.

A second theme is that X-rays allow us to see what should be hidden. This 'invisible light' shows many things, including things that should be revealed such as fractures and diseases; however, there is also a sense that other things revealed are best kept hidden. For example, the

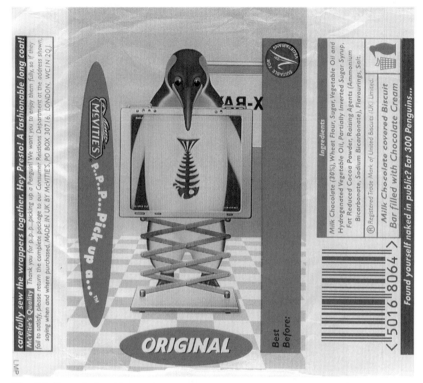

Fig. 4.3 Penguin Bar: X-ray set.

Reproduced with the kind permission of United Biscuits.

customs officer can look for contraband using X-rays and perhaps the husband can check up on his straying wife.

The third theme is the purely educational. Several trade cards illustrated X-ray apparatus and techniques. These cards looks more like an illustration from a contemporary textbook of radiography than something designed to encourage the purchase of chocolate. The images on the cards were not always accurate.

A fourth theme is the X-rays as being naughty and revealing intimate details. There is a cartoon from 1899 illustrating a metal dress for ladies to wear to avoid being viewed by X-rays. The mechanical post card 'X STRAHLEN' has a lever to pull. The postcard starts with a demure and properly dressed couple on a beach. As the lever is pulled the X-rays are applied and the clothes are removed leaving the couple in their swimming costumes! Sometimes the intimate details are unwanted.

The young man presents his fiancé with one of the new Roentgen photographs and she is not at all happy with the skeletal result. The X-rays have revealed more than she had anticipated

A final theme is the look into the future. The card Verbesserte Röntgenstrahlen im Jahre 2000 (Figure 4.4) shows a policeman looking through a wall with an X-ray machine to see the safe breakers and is accompanied by a charming poem:

Stop, who is going to break in in my house?
Thought that Rentier Reichenstein
Than my safe is creaking very much at all
Quick, get the X-rays!
These are so wonderful,
Everything one could see clearly
Through a metre thick wall
The thieves are recognized
Quick he goes to the police
Which comes 1 2 3
Before the rogues can notice
In shackle they are brought.
(Translation by Dr Uwe Busch)

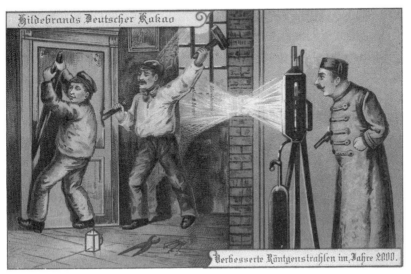

Fig. 4.4 Verbesserte Röntgenstrahlen im Jahre 2000. [A Vision of the Future.] The police using X-rays to show the criminals.

Card published by Hildebrand German Cocoa, c.1900. Image courtesy of Adrian M.K. Thomas.

Radiology and art

Radiographic techniques for analysing paintings came into use soon after Roentgen's discovery[7] and A.W. Konig of Frankfurt is believed to have used X-rays to examine oil paintings shortly after the discovery.

Radiology can be used to authenticate antiques, and in addition radiographic techniques have been used to analyse paintings—to help with dating them and to identify the artists. X-ray analysis of paintings is particularly valuable in oil on canvas images. Analysis of paintings enables the discovery of fakes and fraudulent transactions in the art market and also enables further analysis and understanding of the mechanisms at work in the paintings of the great masters. Recently in March 2012, Louis Van Tilborgh, the curator of research at the Van Gogh museum in Amsterdam, has used X-ray analysis (macro scanning X-ray fluorescence spectometry) of paintings to uncover an unattributed painting of Van Gogh entitled *Still life with flower and roses*. The analysis confirmed the brush strokes and a pigment used by Vincent Van Gogh and thus has led to a new discovery of a painting previously thought to have been painted by someone else. X-ray analysis also helped identify another painting of two wrestlers painted underneath the one of the still life and roses. This painting had been in the possession of the Kröller-Müller Museum in Otterlo, Holland and had not previously been thought to be a Van Gogh original.

X-ray diffraction and spectroscopic techniques have also been used to study the paintings of Vincent Van Gogh, and to explain why the paintings have changed in colour over the years. A team from Antwerp used the X-ray beam generator at the European Synchrotron Radiation Facility in Grenoble, France and analysed the paints and chrome pigments used in Van Gogh paintings to see why they have darkened and concluded that the chrome pigments darkened due to contamination with barium sulphate and ultraviolet light. This is why paintings with chrome yellow should be stored away from strong or ultraviolet light.

The use of X-rays themselves to create beautiful images of objects of course is nothing new and John Hall-Edwards, a Birmingham Radiologist, was using this particular technique almost a hundred years ago and published a paper on X-ray imaging of flowers in 1914 entitled

'The radiography of flowers' and used X-rays to create artistic images of flowers (Figure 4.5).[8] Engelbrecht and Tasker in the 1930s rekindled interest in X-raying flowers to create images and today some of Tasker's original pieces are sought after items.

Film directors have dabbled with radiographic imaging—for example, Roger Corman in his science fiction cult classic film from 1963, *X: The Man with the X-Ray Eyes*.[9] The film, whose protagonist could see through objects, is notable for its early depiction of radiographic images of bodies and buildings and may have inspired subsequent generations of creators of radiographic art. The lobby card showed Dr Xavier having the drops that gives him X-ray vision being instilled into his eyes.

In 1990, a retired professor of dentistry, Albert Richards from Michigan, USA, published a book of flower prints entitled *The Secret*

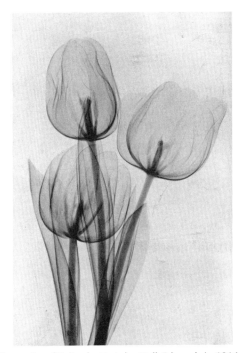

Fig. 4.5 The Radiography of Tulips by Dr John Hall-Edwards in 1914.

Reproduced from Hall-Edwards, The radiography of flowers, *Archives of the Roentgen Ray*, 1914; *19*, pp. 30–31, Copyright © 1914 *British Journal of Radiology*. Image courtesy of the archive of the British Institute of Radiology.

Garden, and in 1994 William Conklin published an entire book on the radiographs of mollusc shells, an object that lends itself to the creation of beautiful X-ray images.

In the past decade or so the application of X-ray techniques to create works of art has become more widespread, with Nick Veasey's recent radiographic images of objects in particular coming to mind. Veasey,[10] a British photographer, used simple X-rays to see through the surface of everyday objects, such as cups and saucers, shoes, and computers, to reveal their inner beauty. This technique pushed the boundaries of photographic art. Leaves and flowers, insects, and fish were displayed as never before. Even large objects such as an aeroplane were X-rayed for the creation of a spectacular radiographic artistic image.

Franz Fellner, an Austrian radiologist from Linz, has recently used cross-sectional imaging techniques including computed tomography (CT) and magnetic resonance imaging (MRI) scanning and with powerful post-processing software has created interesting images of both the body's vascular system as well as musical instruments to create works of art that have been displayed in museums—his ARS INTRINSICA exhibition was on display at the Leopold Museum in Vienna in 2009 and at the Röntgen Museum in Remscheid, Germany, in 2010.

Some other artists using X-rays to create their art include Hugh Turvey, Leslie Wright, Stephen Meyers M.C. Raikes,[11] and Albert Koetsier, all of whom who seem to have taken inspiration from the German and Swiss artist Paul Klee's dictum that art is not about reproducing what we can already see but about making visible that which we cannot.

Radiology and the cinema

It is a somewhat strange coincidence that within a few weeks of Roentgen's discovery of X-rays on 8 November 1895, another major invention involving imaging which was to transform modern 20th-century culture and entertainment was unleashed on the world in Paris by the Lumière brothers who showed their cinematic films for the first time to a paying audience at the Grand Café in the Boulevard du Capucines on 28 December 1895. Within 3 years Lumière had shot or produced over 1000 films and is considered by many to be the father of cinema.

The early silent films were made primarily for entertainment. However, the subject of X-rays had crept into the movies as early as 1897 with the production of commercial silent films *The X-ray Friend* and *The X-ray Mirror* in 1899.

With the advent of the talking pictures in the late 1920s, storytelling evolved more sophisticated themes and not surprisingly medical themes and issues gradually found their way into many films produced in this era. One of the earliest famous films produced of medical and scientific interest was the 1936 film *The story of Louis Pasteur* about the famous French microbiologist. In 1936 a film entitled *The Invisible Ray* starring Boris Karloff dealt with the topic of the harmful effects of radiation for the first time. The film tells the story of a scientist who visits Africa and gets exposed to toxic radiation from a meteorite and has to be saved by an antidote.

In 1943 the lives of the Curies were made into an excellent and very popular film (based on Eve Curie's biography of her mother Marie) starring Greer Garson and Walter Pidgeon. This film *Madam Curie* went on to be nominated for seven Oscars but unfortunately lost out to the much loved masterpiece *Casablanca* starring Humphrey Bogart and Ingrid Bergman, also produced that year.

In 1950 Akira Kurosawa, the Japanese master of cinema, directed a film entitled *Ikiru*. Ikiru means to live. The film was about a man dying of gastric cancer that reassesses his life following his diagnosis and impending death. This was one of the first films to depict a barium meal and a gastric cancer within the barium meal plates can be detected in the scenes.

The 1960s saw further interest in X-ray and radiology in general. They were seen within the spectrum of science fiction. Perhaps the most memorable film of this genre was the 1963 Roger Corman cult classic *The Man with X-ray Eyes*. Ray Milland plays the part of Dr Xavier, a man able to see through objects and people. This film served to bring the science of radiology and X-rays to the public eye. It is interesting to note that Ray Milland had previously played the part of a nuclear scientist and spy in a little remembered 1952 film *The Thief*, made by Russell Rouse and shot without any dialogue.

A further interesting work of science fiction was produced in 1966 entitled *Fantastic Voyage*. This film was notable for the depiction of the interior of the vascular system of the body. The patient has a stroke and a miniaturized vessel is inserted into the bloodstream to navigate its way around to the brain. This was science fiction indeed and was in fact the precursor of interventional radiology, as we know it in the 21st century. Today intravenous vascular procedures and intravenous vascular cameras are no longer the stuff of science fiction and intravascular therapies are commonplace. This film was remade in1987 as *Inner Space* with Dennis Quaid but little in the way of medical imaging was portrayed in this film.

Interventional neuroradiology was depicted in all its blood and gore in a realistic format in William Friedkin's 1973 film *The Exorcist*, based in Washington, DC. The investigation of the brain with carotid puncture was depicted realistically for the first time, albeit it a cult horror movie. The George Washington University was in fact the third site in the USA to receive a CT scanner after the Mayo Clinic and Massachusetts General Hospital in Boston.

Perhaps the most amusing depiction of CT scanning was in the Woody Allen's film *Hannah and Her Sisters*. Woody Allen is shown undergoing a CT scan of his brain. He plays the part of a neurotic who thinks he has brain cancer and the film depicts realistically the process of CT scanning and CT scans of the brain as never depicted before. In 1988 *Hannah and Her Sisters* was to win Woody Allen an Oscar.

More recently radiology and scanning have been depicted in the cinema in futuristic settings such as in the film *Total Recall* in which a giant X-ray machine scans subway passengers. This film was made in 1990 starring Arnold Schwarzenegger and set the standard for computer-generated imaging which was to become almost a part of routine practice in films of the 21st century.

In the 1991 movie *The Doctor*, William Hurt plays the part of a doctor who develops throat cancer. The film shows Hurt undergoing an MRI scan and depicts the real-life anxieties patients undergo while awaiting tests and their subsequent results and consequences.

The 1990s also saw the depiction of real obstetric ultrasound imaging in the movies, notably in *Nine Months* and *Father of the Bride 2*, both released in 1995.

Over the last two decades more and more realistic depictions of medical and health issues have been creeping into mainstream movies and this trend is likely to continue as the world's population ages and become bigger healthcare consumers than ever before.

References

1. **Rickards, M.** (1998). *Collecting Printed Ephemera*. Oxford: Phaidon.
2. **Rickards, M.** (2000). *The Encyclopaedia of Ephemera*. London: The British Library.
3. **Thomas, A.M.K. and Mould, R.F.** (2004). X-ray ephemera, with particular reference to apparatus. *Current Oncology, 11*, 14–33.
4. **Thomas, A.M.K., Busch, U., and Tombach, B.** (2005). Nur einen tag lang—ephemera aus der radiologie. In Bautz, W. and Busch, U. (Eds), *100 Jahre Deutsche Röntgengesellschaft*, pp. 124–127. Stuttgart: Thieme Verlag.
5. **Howsden, G.** (1995). *Collecting Cigarette and Trade Cards*. London: New Cavendish Books.
6. **Steff, F.** (1966). *The Picture Postcard and its Origins*. London: Lutterworth Press.
7. **Banerjee, A.K.** (2011). Inside art—review of the week. *British Medical Journal, 342*, d240.
8. **Hall-Edwards, J.** (1914). The radiography of flowers. *Archives of the Roentgen Ray, 19*, 30–31.
9. **Banerjee, A.K.** (2008). Review of the week: the man with X-ray eyes. *British Medical Journal, 336*, 1193.
10. **Veasey, N.** (2008). *X-Ray. Nick Veasey. See Through The World Around You*. London: Carlton Books.
11. **Raikes, M.C.** (2003). Floral radiography – using X-rays to create fine art. *RadioGraphics, 23*, 1149–1154.

Chapter 5

Classical radiology

The plain film

The medical applications of radiography were apparent immediately, however in the early years of radiography the apparatus was of a low power and it was difficult to see through the thicker parts of the body.[1] This was particularly the case with plain film radiography; however, fluoroscopy was more effective and was used for examining the chest and thick parts of the body. The cryptoscope is a simple fluorescent screen which is covered by a lightproof hood with eyeholes so that the screen can be observed. Figure 5.1 is from *The ABC of the X-rays* written by William Meadowcroft in 1896. It shows a radiographer using a cryptoscope to examine his own hand. The cryptoscope was often used to test the quality of the X-ray tube and the hand was a convenient object and this is one reason for the high incidence of injuries to the hand with early X-ray workers. The cryptoscope was used quite widely until the 1940s and gradually passed out of use. Versions were made for surgeons that could be strapped to the head leaving both hands free for operating.

In his book Meadowcroft discusses how coins and dense structures will block the passage of X-rays and says that:

> The same effect will be produced by placing the hand in front of the screen, and pressed tightly on the outside of the screen, and in front of the tube. The rays would pass through the flesh, blood, sinews and muscles, but the bones being opaque, their shadows would be cast upon the screen. Of course, there is no permanent shadow left upon the screen by placing any objects in front of it as above-mentioned. As soon as the generation of X-rays ceases, there is, of course, nothing to cause the crystals to exhibit fluorescence, and the screen will, therefore, become dark. It is evident, therefore, that the fluoroscope is a device which can be used indefinitely if properly taken care of.[2]

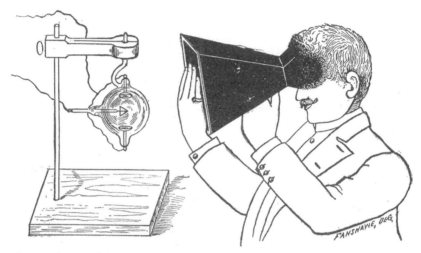

Fig. 5.1 The use of the cryptoscope. Note the unprotected X-ray tube and the operator's hand used as a test object.

Reproduced from William Henry Meadowcroft, *The A B C of the X rays*, The American Technical Book Co., USA, Copyright © 1896. Image courtesy of Dr Adrian M.K. Thomas.

Wilhelm Röntgen, when he discovered X-rays in 1895, described both their effects on a fluorescent screen and on photographic glass and therefore described both radiography and fluoroscopy.

By the end of the 19th century photography was well developed, and images could be recorded on glass plates, film, and paper. In England Frederick Scott Archer had invented the wet collodion process for coating glass plates with silver salts in 1851; however, its disadvantage was that the collodion had to remain wet on the plate during both exposure and developing. This was improved in 1871 when Richard Maddox invented the gelatin silver bromide dry glass plate, which had the advantage that the gelatin could dry on the glass plate. The glass plates had to be coated by hand until 1879 when George Eastman, who founded Kodak, invented a machine process. In 1889 George Eastman introduced flexible transparent photographic film made of cellulose nitrate, which was unfortunately highly flammable but made roll film possible. In 1913 Kodak introduced a specialized X-ray film but still on a cellulose nitrate base. Much of the photographic glass was made in Belgium and conditions during the First World War made supply of the glass difficult. The demand for X-rays also increased and therefore radiographs glass plates gradually passed out of use and by the 1920s film was used almost universally. It is interesting to observe that even in the 1990s before picture archiving and communication systems (PACS) and digital imaging it was common to see on an X-ray request form the letters WPP when the patient was to return to the clinic with the unreported films. WPP stood for 'Wet Plates Please', which was amusing since wet plates had not been available since before the First World War! In PACS the digital radiographic image is stored on a computer archive and viewed on a screen as a soft copy.

In 1923 Kodak introduced cellulose acetate as a base for the film and this was marketed as safety film. Sadly this did not prevent the tragedy at the Cleveland Clinic in Ohio on 15 May 1929.There was an explosion in the X-ray department when escaping steam from a leaking pipe ignited the X-ray film store, which exploded and sent a cloud of poisonous fumes through the building. The explosion rocked the building and the blinding smoke and intense heat hindered the work of the firefighters. Many of those who were rescued had their faces stained yellow by the fumes and subsequently died from smoke inhalation. A total of 126 died in what must be the worst disaster affecting an X-ray department in peacetime. The early film was made of cellulose nitrate, which was highly flammable.

The traditional manual processing of radiographs was gradually automated and in 1942 Pako introduced the first automatic film processor. The initial automatic processors replicated the manual process until Kodak introduced the first roller transport film processor in 1956. Darkrooms were replaced as daylight processing was introduced and 3M introduced the first laser imager in 1984. 3M introduced a dry-processor laser imaging system in 1994. Modern departments now use no film at all and only CDs are printed if required at all, with most image transmissions between hospitals taking place via image links.

Conventional tomography

The problem with conventional radiography is that the radiographic image is a two-dimensional shadow of a three-dimensional structure.[3]

Before the computed tomography (CT) scanner there were several techniques used to obtain depth information. One was stereoscopy with two images taken with a tube shift to give a three-dimensional image, the principle upon which rangefinders were used for military purposes and for focusing in rangefinder cameras including Leica and Voightlander, especially before the days of through-the-lens focusing. This technique was available with conventional photography at the time Röntgen made his discovery. Alternatively two images could be recorded on a single film with a tube shift, and using a parallax technique the depth of a foreign body could be measured. The other technique is tomography, which is a means of examining separate planes in a structure by blurring out features that are not in the plane of interest. In this simple technique the patient stays still and the X-ray tube and film move about an axis. The technique of conventional tomography had been developed independently by several workers in the 1920s starting with André Bocage in 1921. There were many solutions to the problem of tomography with work by Ziedes des Plantes, Jean Kieffer, and others. In December 1935 G. Grossmann from Berlin described his well-known tomogram. Edward W. Twining from Manchester developed a simple tomographic attachment to an X-ray table, which he described in April 1937. One of Vallebona's techniques was to keep the tube stationary and move the patient and film. The problem could be solved by a variety of methods and in 1937 the British radiographer William Watson built his apparatus in which the patient was upright and rotated. The images obtained were therefore axial tomograms and resembled CT slices.

The apparatus used was elegant and instead of simple planar shift could use complex movements such as hypocycloidal for fine tomography of the inner ear. Tomography persisted for some time after the introduction of the CT scanner. There were several reasons for this including familiarity with the technique and poor resolution in the early generations of the CT scanner. The only current use for conventional tomography is its occasional use in the kidney during intravenous pyelography and even this is gradually fading away.

The gastrointestinal tract

Following Röntgen's discovery, the application of X-rays to investigating the skeleton was soon realized but it was not initially thought that the application would be much use in the gastrointestinal tract. In the years before modern endoscopy barium studies were central to examination of the gastrointestinal tract.[4]

Early attempts to image the abdomen were unsuccessful because the weak X-rays produced were unable to penetrate the soft tissue. However, Wegele suggested that a stomach tube should be placed in the patient with a wire placed through it and by this means the dimensions of the stomach would be obtained. The first published pictures of this technique, however, were produced by Lindemann a year later in 1897. The real major breakthrough in gastrointestinal radiology came with the discovery of bismuth as a suitable contrast agent. A Philadelphian, George E. Pfahler (1874–1957) noted in 1897 that a photographic plate of a patient's abdomen showed bismuth in the stomach. Bismuth used to be a remedy for gastric ulcers at the turn of the century. The observations were followed up by another pioneering radiologist from Philadelphia, Charles L. Leonard (1861–1913) and also by two Frenchmen, Roux and Balthazard, who mixed bismuth with liquid and solid food to study the movements of the stomach.

Around this time a first year medical student at Harvard Medical School (later to become a professor) named Walter B. Cannon began a research project with a fellow student, Moser. The project had been suggested by Bowditch who was a Professor of Physiology at that time. The students performed experiments studying deglutition with X-rays using bismuth capsules. They studied deglutition in dogs, frogs, and cats and presented their work before the American Physiological Society. They studied gastric movements and Cannon observed 'The stomach movements are inhibited whenever the cat shows signs of anxiety, rage or distress'.[4] Cannon eventually studied gastric movements in humans and collaborated with Francis H. Williams in the study of oesophageal and stomach movement in children. Williams was a respected Boston physician who in 1901 produced an important 658-page textbook

The Roentgen Rays in Medicine and Surgery. Pioneering work in gastrointestinal imaging was also being conducted in Europe. In Germany, Hermann Rieder (1885–1932) published a paper describing the bismuth meal and advocated rapid serial filming, a forerunner of the modern barium meal. In Vienna in 1905 Guido Hotzknecht (1872–1931), a future radiation martyr, advocated fluoroscopic examination of the gastrointestinal tract.

Back in New York, Lewis G. Idle (1874–1954), the innovative American radiologist, built up a vast experience using the Rieder method, whereas at the Mayo Clinic, Russell D. Carman (1875–1926), a follower of the Viennese School built up a vast experience of fluoroscopic investigations resulting in probably the first book on gastrointestinal radiology.

British pioneers included Alfred E. Barclay (1876–1949) (whose name has been given to a medal awarded by the British Institute of Radiology) who preferred a combination of screen and plate methods in the investigation of the upper gastrointestinal tract. A review of the radiology literature would be incomplete without mentioning the pioneering Swedish School of Radiology. Radiology began in 1905 in Sweden thanks mainly to the pioneering anatomist Gösta Forssell who undertook scientific studies on the stomach and duodenum. In addition, he was founder editor of *Acta Radiolgica*, was involved in the planning of the Karolinska Institute, and trained Lysholm and Lindgren, who both subsequently became pioneering neuroradiologists in their own right.

The early part of the 20th century resulted in workers concentrating primarily on the upper gastrointestinal tract. Figure 5.2 shows a penetrating gastric ulcer (arrowed) on an opaque meal in 1917. However, it was not long before the colon became an organ of interest. Schule probably first described a contrast investigation of the large bowel using bismuth and oil enema to image the colon in 1904. Initial studies were all single-contrast studies. The value of double-contrast studies for studying mucosal detail, however, had been recognized as early as 1906 by Holzknecht who used an effervescent agent for studying the stomach. The first double-contrast enema was described by Laurell of Uppsala in 1921. By this time bismuth was found to be toxic and had been replaced

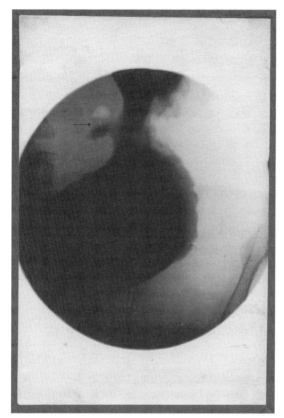

Fig. 5.2 Gastric ulcer (arrowed) on an opaque meal from 1917.
Image donated by the Scott Family. Reproduced courtesy of Dr Adrian M.K. Thomas.

by barium. Fischer in Frankfurt refined the technique of air insuffla-
tion and, following a visit by Kirklin in 1928, the technique was brought
into use at the Mayo Clinic. The technique became firmly established
following the publications by Welin in Malmo, Sweden, who showed
that polyps could be demonstrated in 12.5% of all patients. Back in
England, Young introduced a modification of the Malmo enema at
St Mark's Hospital whereas Miller of Indiana University popularized the method in the USA. The Japanese too were great enthusiasts
of the double-contrast technique following the pioneering studies of
Shirakabe who used the double-contrast enema study of the colon to
study the pathology of intestinal tuberculosis. With the improvement

in barium suspensions and effervescent agents, double-contrast studies of both the lower and upper gastrointestinal tracts have become routine. Diagnostic imaging of the small bowel was not really possible until the development of flocculation-resistant barium suspensions in the 1950s. Pioneers included Golden who favoured a small volume of oral barium (250ml) and Marshak who favoured larger volumes of 500ml to 600ml.

The first person to describe a technique of duodenal intubation was Pesquera in 1929. It was Schatzki, however, who coined the term small intestinal enema in 1943, reporting on 75 cases. This method of investigating the mucosal detail of the small bowel has been modified by several workers including the British radiologist Scott-Harden who is notable for the introduction of the coaxial tube for easier duodenal intubation. Sellink in America has popularized his single-contrast enteroclysis technique using a modified Bilbao–Dotter tube and Gianturco wire. Nolan, the Oxford radiologist, using a transnasal 12-French catheter for duodenal intubation, has simplified the technique.

A historical review of diagnostic imaging of the gastrointestinal tract would be incomplete without at least some mention of endoscopic imaging. Rigid tubes were introduced into the stomach as long ago as 1865 by Kussmaul who used a gastric tube for aspirating the stomach contents of a patient attending his clinic. The semiflexible gastroscope was introduced in 1932 by Schindler (1888–1968) who produced the first book on the subject entitled *Lehrbuch und Atlas der Gastroskopie*. Further advances in instrumentation were made possible with the development of fibreoptic systems by Hopkins and following this fibreoptic flexible instruments were introduced in Japan, the USA, and UK. By the end of the 1960s a colonoscope with a controllable tip became available, enabling the complete colon to be imaged using this technique.

Contrast media and the renal tract

From the earliest days after the discovery of X-rays the rays were used to investigate the renal tract.[5] The low power of the early apparatus made abdominal investigation difficult due to the thickness of the body part and the prolonged radiographic exposure needed. Although abdominal compression devices such as that employed by Henirich Albers-Schönberg (1865–1921) in Germany were helpful, it was only following the development of more powerful apparatus that more meaningful images could be obtained. The radiographic shadow pictures or skiagrams were confusing to the early investigators and it was difficult to define the nature of calcification in lymph nodes, fibroids, calculi, calcified tuberculosis, and phleboliths.

Using the cystoscope it was possible to introduce a ureteric catheter, which could be followed by abdominal radiography. This was first done by Schmidt and Kolischer independently in 1901, having been suggested by Tuffier in 1898. In 1908 Hurry Fenwick from the Royal London Hospital produced his classic book *The Value of Radiography in the Diagnosis and Treatment of Urinary Stone*. In 1905 Fenwick had introduced bougies with their wall impregnated with radio-opaque metal into the ureters, and radiography could show their course and the location of calculi. In 1897 he had also used a small fluorescent screen (the cryptoscope) to examine diseased kidneys at the time of operative surgery. Fenwick was a remarkable man and was an early exponent of the correlation of the clinical, radiological, and pathological features of disease.

The use of bougies and catheters was soon followed by the injection of radio-opaque material into the renal tract as suggested by Klose in 1904. For retrograde pyelography, a suspension of bismuth subnitrate was used but the method was difficult and it was awkward to remove the bismuth from the renal tract. The technique of retrograde pyelography was refined by Voelcker and von Lichtenberg in 1906 and they produced the first complete outline of the ureter and renal pelvis. They used a 2% solution of collargol (colloidal silver) but the technique was not without problems that were related to the difficulty in inserting ureteric catheters and the toxicity of the agents used (Figure 5.3). These silver-based compounds were toxic to the kidneys and when excessive pressure was used for injection they sometimes resulted in fatal renal necrosis. In the USA Braasch investigated these compounds extensively, demonstrating areas of renal necrosis.

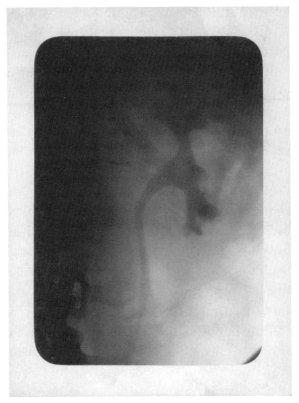

Fig. 5.3 Collargol in the renal pelvis in a retrograde pyelogram.
Image donated by the Scott Family. Reproduced courtesy of Dr Adrian M.K. Thomas.

These severe toxic effects demonstrated the need for safer contrast agents. In 1907 Burkhardt and Polano injected oxygen into the renal pelvis as a negative contrast agent but the radiographic shadow was difficult to distinguish from bowel gas. In 1915 thorium salts were used but a major advance was made in 1918 when a young surgeon, Douglas Cameron of Minnesota, recommended the use of sodium and potassium iodide for retrograde pyelography.

Following the successful introduction of retrograde pyelography, von Lichtenberg who was Professor of Urology at St Hedwick's Hospital in Berlin, undertook extensive laboratory work in an attempt to develop clinical intravenous urography but without success. The nearest approach to a successful intravenous urogram (IVU) was achieved by Hryntschalk of Vienna in 1929 who succeeded in producing good radiographic visualization of the renal calyces and pelvises in laboratory animals after intravenous injection of iodinated pyridine compounds probably synthesized by Binz and Räth, but he did not disclose the nature of the products and his work was not fully accepted by the medical establishment.

In 1923 a team of workers at the Mayo Clinic, Osborne (a syphilologist), Scholl (a urologist), Sutherland (a radiologist), and Rowntree (a physician), described the use of intravenous and oral sodium iodide to visualize the urinary tract. Osborne had noticed that the urinary bladder was visible on radiographs of patients taking large doses of oral and intravenous sodium iodide for the treatment of syphilis. The visualization of the renal pelvis was poor but the authors calibrated the dose of iodine against the urinary iodine concentration and the degree of bladder radio-opacity. However, sodium iodide was far too toxic for clinical radiodiagnosis.

In 1925 and 1926 Arthur Binz and Curt Räth who were professors of chemistry from the Agricultural College in Berlin synthesized many organic iodine and arsenical preparations based on the pyridine ring in an attempt to produce an improved drug for the treatment of syphilis and other infections. The pyridine ring is a six-pointed ring made up of five carbon atoms and one nitrogen atom. Linkage to this ring greatly detoxified the arsenic and iodine atoms. Binz and Räth synthesized more than 700 of these compounds. One group of iodinated pyridine compounds was found to be excreted selectively by the liver and kidney and was therefore called the 'selectans'. Some of these synthesized pyridine drugs were sent to several clinicians for evaluation for the treatment of gall bladder and kidney infections.

In 1928, Moses Swick (1900–1985), who was working as a urology intern at Mount Sinai Hospital in New York, was awarded the Libman Scholarship encouraging medical research overseas. He went to work with Professor Leopold Lichtwitz at the Altona Krankenhaus in Hamburg, Germany, where he had some success in the treatment of human biliary coccal infections with some of Binz and Räth's iodinated selectan drugs. Since these drugs contained iodine, it occurred to Swick that they might be of value in visualizing the renal tract by radiography.

Swick made radiological, chemical, and toxicological studies in laboratory animals and patients. The initial studies were encouraging and Swick transferred his work to gain access to the large number of patients at the urological department of Professor Alexander von Lichtenberg at St Hedwig's Hospital in Berlin. The first successful human IVUs were produced with (non-ionic) N-methyl-5-iodo-2 pyridone (selectan neutral) but Swick preferred the less toxic, more soluble salt 5-iodo-2-pyridone-N-acetate sodium (uroselectan) that had been patented by Räth in May 1927. This new compound uroselectan produced excellent quality IVUs with relatively little toxicity and thereafter the practice of urology was changed forever.

Swick and von Lichtenberg presented the work to the Ninth Congress of the German Urological Society in September 1929, with Swick presenting the first paper based on the animal work but with several excellent quality human studies exhibiting various disease processes (e.g. hydronephrosis and horseshoe kidney). Von Lichtenberg and Swick together presented the second paper on the human clinical uses with the paper read by von Lichtenberg. The two papers were published in November 1929 in *Klinische Wochenschrift.*

Unfortunately Swick and von Lichtenberg could not agree on who should be accorded priority of discovery of this revolutionary diagnostic technique which excited the medical world. Von Lichtenberg felt that he, as the senior professor, should be the principal author of the new method as his patients and laboratories had been used and his links with Binz and Räth had been very helpful in supplying the contrast agents. But von Lichtenberg had been on an extended lecture tour in America when Swick had undertaken the research and had produced the first ever successful and reliable human IVUs. The young inexperienced Swick was determined that he (who had devised and conducted the urographic research) should be accorded the accolade of primacy of discovery rather than the distinguished professor.

Swick returned to the USA for the June 1930 meeting of the American Urological association in New York. Intravenous urography was the primary topic and Alexander von Lichtenberg was the guest of honour, presenting the first American paper. Moses Swick was not even invited and, despite his urgent pleas, was not even permitted to attend. The dispute between Swick and von Lichtenberg continued. Lichwitz strongly supported Swick in his claim as the originator of the technique of intravenous urography, while Binz and Räth strongly supported von Lichtenberg. The medical establishment accepted the distinguished von Lichtenberg as the real originator and Swick was regarded as a very junior assistant, a plagiarist, and a cheat and he was shunned by the international medical community.

Swick continued to work as a urologist at Mount Sinai Hospital, New York, but for 35 years he practised under the cloud of deceit. Following Victor Marshall's investigation, in 1966 Moses Swick was awarded the Valentine Medal of the American Academy of Medicine and was recognized as the real developer of the IVU. The American Congressional Record of 16 May 1978 stated that Swick's work was 'one of the five major contributions of an individual to medicine'.[5] These ionic and high-osmolar contrast media were very successful and with modifications were the standard intravascular and urologic contrast media until the 1970s. Their use was not without complications and they were irritant, caused a severe sense of warmth when injected, and patients often vomited.

Torsten Almén and low-osmolar contrast media

Torsten Almén (b. 1931) (Figure 5.4), who as a young Swedish radiologist was working at Malmö, studied the pharmacology of contrast agents and considered that the very high osmolality of high-osmolality contrast media (up to eight times physiological osmolality, 300mOsmol per kilogram of water) was responsible for much of its toxicity. Almén grew up on the most southern coast of Sweden and recalls a holiday as a boy in Bohuslän on the west coast of Sweden. He found swimming in the water uncomfortable because as soon as he opened his eyes they started to hurt. The salty water at Bohuslän made his eyes sore whereas the brackish water around Ystad did not cause discomfort. He reasoned that 'a plasma-isotonic aqueous solution of contrast medium molecules might not cause pain, and should therefore be created!'[5]

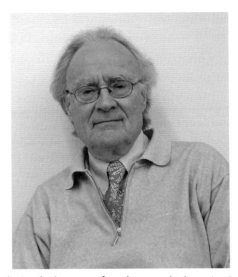

Fig. 5.4 Torsten Almén, the inventor of modern non-ionic contrast media.

Reproduced from Thomas, A.M.K., Banerjee, A.K., and Busch, U. (Eds.) *Classic Papers in Modern Diagnostic Radiology*, 2005, Springer Berlin Heidelberg with permission from Torsten Almén.

Almén taught himself the relevant chemistry and suggested reducing the osmolality of contrast media by substituting the non-radio-opaque cation by a non-ionizing radical such as an amide. His paper on this topic was prepared when he was a Research Fellow in Philadelphia in 1968 to 1969. His thesis, completely theoretical and unsupported by chemical or clinical research, was rejected by the leading radiological journals but was eventually accepted and published by the *Journal of Theoretical Biology* in 1969, a journal of which most radiologists were unaware. Thus the most important paper on contrast media since Swick's 1929 paper was lost to the radiological publications.

Almén's ideas were rejected by several pharmaceutical manufacturers but Hugo Holterman, the Research Director of Nyegaard,[6] encouraged his team to attempt synthesis of some of Almén's theoretical molecules. It is remarkable that fewer than 6 months were to elapse between the first meeting of Almén and the Nyegaard research group in June 1968 and the production of the first compound. A consultant reviewer of Almén's 1969 paper stated: 'The general principles of Dr Almén's proposal is probably sound. The implementation of it is probably impractical. He seems to be unaware that the ionic nature of the iodinated compounds is an essential property for their solubility in water—so part of his proposal, namely using non-ionic hydrophilic compounds, may be invalid'.[6] In November 1969 after biological and pharmacological testing, compound 16 (called 'Sweet Sixteen') was shown to be the most promising and it was marketed as Amipaque (the first low-osmolar contrast medium (LOCM)). Amipaque was based on the glucose amide of Isopaque (metrizoate) leading to its generic name metrizamide (Amipaque). As it contained the glucose radical, metrizamide could not be autoclaved. Because of the complexities of its production, it was expensive and inconvenient to use, being presented as a freeze-dried powder with a diluent. It was, however, a major toxicological improvement on all pre-existing water-soluble myelographic and vascular agents and in the late 1970s it became the internationally recognized agent for myelography, enabling water-soluble myelography to replace oil (Myodil, Pantopaque) myelography. Although it had an advantageous intravascular profile, metrizamide was generally regarded as too expensive and too inconvenient for vascular studies. Deservedly, at the 1989 World Congress of Radiology Torsten Almén was presented with the Antoine Béclère Prize.

A few years later, in the mid-1970s, metrizamide was replaced by the second-generation LOCM Iohexol and Iopamidol which are easier to synthesize and therefore much less expensive. They do not contain the glucose radical, can be autoclaved, and are stable in solution. These two second-generation LOCM, together with similar molecules, remain the contrast media of choice for intravascular procedures in the mid-1990s. This has led the way for intravascular interventional therapy, which has successfully challenged and in several areas replaced conventional surgery. However, we should remember how good the early contrast media were and that the first successful agent was non-ionic.

Traditional neuroradiology

The brain is difficult to investigate and while there might have been a hope that radiology could be of assistance this was not the case until the work of Walter Dandy in 1918 and 1919.[7] The first paper in the journal *Brain* devoted to radiology did not appear until 1924 and the *British Journal of Radiology* did not mention neuroradiology until 1916 when Stenvers wrote about his radiographic views of the orbit.

The major early figure in neuroradiology was Arthur Schüller from Vienna whose book *Röntgendiagnostik der Erkrankungen des Kopfes* was published in 1911. Schüller described many of the classic plain film findings including pineal shift, cranial calcification, and diseases of the pituitary fossa.

Ventriculography and encephalography

There had been several case reports of patients surviving with intracranial air. One such case was described by Sebastian Gilbert Scott in 1915 (Figure 5.5), showing pneumocephaly in a woman who complained of her brain splashing. Walter Dandy from Johns Hopkins Hospital was aware of this and also of the value of abnormal gas collections to diagnose abdominal disease. In 1918 Dandy described ventriculography and in 1919 encephalography. In the latter air is injected at lumbar puncture in order to fill the ventricular system. Dandy also predicted the development of air myelography for spinal lesions, and subsequently this was performed by Jacobaeus from Stockholm who demonstrated three spinal tumours in 1921. Encephalography was not easy and at the first International Congress of Radiology held in London in 1925 J.W. Pierson, who was a colleague of Dandy, said that the procedure was dangerous and complicated, but in favour said that in competent hands it should not be nearly so dangerous as exploratory craniotomy and could give more information. Dandy had three deaths in a series of 500 examinations. Following the description of ventriculography by Dandy in 1918, the neurosurgeon Harvey Cushing reproached him for spoiling the intellectual challenge of deducing the site of the brain lesion from the history and physical examination. Currently the issue is reversed and it has been quipped that the patient is now referred to the neurologist when the CT or magnetic resonance imaging (MRI) scan is normal!

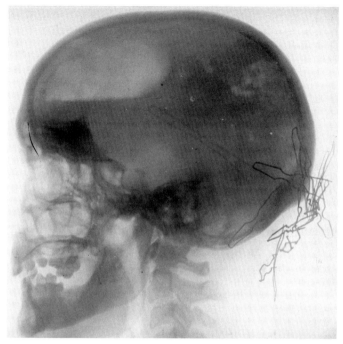

Fig. 5.5 Spontaneous pneumocephaly, a woman whose brain was splashing, 1915.
Image courtesy of Dr Adrian M.K. Thomas.

Myelographic agents

Jean Sicard and Jacques Forestier had been using epidural injections of Lipiodol to treat sciatica and had injected it intrathecally without harm. Lipiodol was used for myelography until iopendylate (Pantopaque or Myodil) was first used in 1944. Iopendylate was not water soluble and was absorbed only slowly. There was a small risk of adhesive arachnoiditis following its use. Before 1970, only iodinated oils including Myodil (Pantopaque) were available for myelography. Ionic compounds were generally considered too toxic although occasionally they were used for lumbosacral radiculography. The ionic water soluble agents Conray and Dimer X were introduced in 1972 and the non-ionic metrizamide in 1977. The French company Guerbet developed the ionic compound meglumine iocarmate (Dimer-X), combining two tri-iodinated benzene rings into one large molecule (hence dimer) containing six atoms of iodine and so reducing the osmolality. Dimer-X could only be used in the lower portions of the spinal canal below the spinal cord for radiculography but it produced superb quality radiographs of the lumbosacral nerve roots. Though much less toxic than the previous aqueous contrast media, it had to be used with great care and in strictly limited dosage. By contrast, metrizamide could be used throughout the spinal canal and was much less toxic than meglumine iocarmate, which it replaced for myelography and radiculography in the late 1970s. Initially metrizamide was limited in use to the thoracolumbar region and until 1980 a special licence was needed from the Department of Health to examine the basal cisterns of the brain. The water-soluble agents showed the nerve root sheaths better and so Myodil was abandoned.

The practice in the UK was to use a smaller quantity of Myodil and to aspirate it after the procedure, which is part of the reason for the lower incidence of adhesive arachnoiditis in the UK. The topic of informed consent of patients before radiological procedures is important. By the 1990s it was good practice to discuss possible side effects and complications with the patient before a radiological procedure but this did not apply during the period of Myodil use. It was generally believed, somewhat paternalistically, that a patient should not be worried unnecessarily by an overemphasis on side effects since he might then refuse a procedure that the doctor believed would be in his best interests.

Angiography

From the earliest days of the application of X-rays, *in vitro* or postmortem angiograms had been used. Direct puncture and/or cut-down arteriography was achieved with sodium iodide and bromide solutions in the early 1920s but the major breakthrough in angiography was achieved in the Santa Marta Hospital in Lisbon, Portugal, on 28 June 1928 when the first successful human carotid arteriogram was performed.[8]

The charismatic leader of the Portuguese team was the professor of neurology, Egas Moniz, a brilliant polymath, author, politician and Portuguese Foreign Secretary, researcher, and clinician. He developed prefrontal leucotomy for which he received the Nobel Prize in Physiology or Medicine in 1949. Moniz was severely handicapped by gout and was unable to make any injections himself, but he meticulously planned his research project on the diagnosis and localization of cerebral tumours. He was dissatisfied with ventriculography, which made a correct diagnosis in less than a third of patients. Initially he thought of opacifying the brain itself by intravenous or parenteral administration. He tried a variety of agents giving large intravenous and parenteral doses of lithium bromide and strontium bromide. After these techniques failed he tried arterial injections using an iodide salt. He chose iodine because of its higher atomic weight compared to bromine. After many difficulties he was successful and his technique involved a 25% solution of sodium iodide with bilateral carotid artery cut-downs. His successful patient, on 28 June 1927, was the ninth in his series, a young man with a pituitary tumour.

Moniz's surgical colleague Reynaldo dos Santos, professor of surgery in Lisbon, in 1929 introduced percutaneous aortography by direct aortic puncture with injection of sodium iodide solution. Translumbar aortography remained a standard for vascular imaging until the 1980s. Other members of Moniz's team were equally innovative and successfully introduced pulmonary angiography (de Carvalho and Almeida Lima), lymphography (Monteiro), phlebography (Joäo Cid des Santos (son of Reynaldo)), and portal venography (Pereira). The Portuguese School therefore introduced many aspects of clinical angiography in the period from 1930 to 1950 but the international adoption of their techniques was severely delayed by the Second World War.

The techniques of neuroradiology developed as the 1930s progressed. Full air encephalography was a major procedure and was not to be undertaken without proper indications. The main exponent of encephalography was Eric Lysholm from Stockholm and he was a master of the technique. The neuroradiology department at the National Hospital for Nervous Diseases in Queen Square was named in his honour. The technique developed and Edward Wing Twining from Manchester gave a masterly Hunterian Lecture in 1936 on the radiology of the third and fourth ventricles and devised a mercury model used to show the problems of filling the third ventricle. In 1937 Hugh Davies from Queen Square described his use of cerebral angiography and for this technique he used a colloidal suspension of dioxide of thorium (Thorotrast) injected directly into the carotid artery. Thorotrast gave beautiful images but had the disadvantage of not being excreted from the body and being radioactive resulting in an incidence of radiation-induced malignancy including angiosarcoma.

By the 1940s the pioneer neuroradiologist Arthur Schüller was working at the Nuffield Institute for Medical Research in Oxford and was investigating the subarachnoid cisterns and their demonstration using a positive contrast agent.

In the post-war period E. Lindgren from Stockholm was perfecting his technique for direct puncture percutaneous cerebral angiography. Encephalography and angiography became standard techniques for the investigation of intracranial pathology. Specialist apparatus was developed to perform these techniques. It might be expected that clinicians would greet the introduction of these procedures with enthusiasm but 20 years after the introduction of cerebral angiography James Bull from the National Hospital for Nervous Diseases in Queen Square was still finding it difficult to submit patients to the procedure. When a Swedish radiologist (presumably Lindgren) who was performing 400 angiograms each year gave a lecture at Queen Square a neurologist commented, 'Those Swedes cannot begin to know their clinical neurology. How could they possibly justify all those cerebral angiograms. It is monstrous'.[9] Following this, cerebral angiography became established in the UK and was usually performed under general anaesthesia. It would be interesting to interview that neurologist today and ask him how current knowledge of clinical neurology influences contemporary referral fates for MRI and CT of the brain which is several orders of magnitude greater than the number of patients who were referred for traditional neuroimaging.

The techniques in the period before CT and MRI reached a remarkable degree of sophistication. For example, in 1970 Glyn Lloyd from Moorefield's Eye Hospital was investigating proptosis using plain films, conventional tomography, subtraction macro-angiography, and contrast orbitography, orbital pneumography, and orbital venography. Orbital pneumography showed the optic nerve elegantly by radiography following the retrobulbar injection of air. The subtraction angiography was made using a photographic technique originally devised by Ziedes des Plantes. Most of these traditional techniques that required a high degree of radiological and radiographic skill for performing and interpreting the results have been replaced by cross-sectional imaging and are being forgotten.

Chest imaging including the tuberculosis screening story

The first book in English devoted to chest radiography was written by G. Harrison Orton and Hugh Walsham and published in 1906 as *The Röntgen Rays in the Diagnosis of Diseases of the Chest*. Even by 1906 there was a huge improvement compared to the 1890s and they were able to assert that 'In the diagnosis of thoracic aneurysm the X-rays reach one of their most successful practical applications. The diagnosis by the ordinary methods is in many cases extremely difficult and in some absolutely impossible; with the aid of the Röntgen rays, however, a satisfactory conclusion can as a rule be arrived at'.[10] Part of the problem with radiography is that the rays can show an abnormality in a patient without physical signs or symptoms. This rather changed the traditional concept of disease and it could be difficult for the radiologist to persuade the physician that the patient had tuberculosis as demonstrated by the radiograph. It took several decades for chest radiography to be applied widely and even in 1919 when Sir William Osler succumbed to the effects of an empyema there was no suggestion that he should be radiographed. Unfortunately it is easy to pass from one extreme to another and it was not uncommon in chest clinics in the 1950s and 1960s for patients to have a radiograph on arrival and the film packets became very full in consequence.

The thoroscope was a common item seen in chest clinics in the mid-20th century. It consisted of a simple fluorescent screen and was used for upright fluoroscopy (Figure 5.6). Dark adaptation of the operator's eyes would be required to view the dim image. It was designed as a compact and completely self-contained unit and was recommended for the consulting room of the private physician and in tuberculosis centres. It was very easy to operate but its very ease of use could result

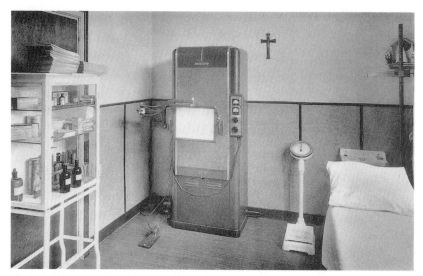

Fig. 5.6 The thorascope, the erect fluoroscopic stand for examination of the chest.
Image courtesy of Dr Adrian M.K. Thomas.

in unnecessary dosage with untoward effects. J.D. Boice and others reviewed the incidence of breast cancer in 4940 women treated for tuberculosis between 1925 and 1954. There were 2573 women examined by X-ray fluoroscopy for an average of 88 times when they had lung collapse therapy for pulmonary tuberculosis. In this group there were 147 breast cancers when only 113.6 were to be expected without an excess of breast cancer in 2367 women treated by other methods. The increased rates for breast cancer were seen from 10 to 15 years after the initial fluoroscopy. The age at exposure strongly influenced the risk of radiation-induced breast cancer with young women being at highest risk and women over 40 being at lowest risk. The mean radiation dosage to the breast was estimated to be 79cGy, and there was strong evidence for a linear relationship between dose and breast cancer risk. It is unfortunate that such an elegant piece of apparatus was associated with such harmful effects.

Kathleen C. Clark and mass miniature radiography

The radiographer K.C. Clark also did pioneering work on the development on mass miniature radiography and the Medical Research Council

Special Report (Series No 251) *Mass Miniature Radiography of Civilians for the Detection of Pulmonary Tuberculosis (Guide to Administration and Technique with a Mobile Apparatus Using 35-mm. Film: And Results of a Survey)* was published in 1945. The authors were Kathleen C. Clark, P. D'Arcy Hart, Peter Kerley, and Brian C. Thompson.

Mass miniature radiography of the chest was being developed in the 1940s. S. Cochrane Shanks was to have given his Presidential Address to the Faculty of Radiologists, which subsequently became the Royal College of Radiologists, in 1940 but because of the conditions of the war it was not formally delivered although it is a most interesting study of mass radiography of the chest. There was considerable interest in mass chest radiography and it was thought useful in examining military recruits, workers in the war industry, and season ticket holders for the public air raid shelters. The main object of mass chest radiography was to detect early pulmonary disease. The technique became more important in the 1950s when effective treatments for pulmonary tuberculosis with drug therapy became more available following clinical trials. There were major antituberculosis campaigns in Scotland in the late 1950s and Figure 5.7 illustrates a badge that was given away in Glasgow. The campaign in the City of Glasgow was held from 11 March to 12 April 1957 and 714,915 persons were X-rayed in 37 units.

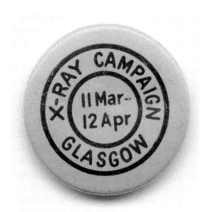

Fig. 5.7 A badge given away in the 1957 Glasgow tuberculosis campaign.
Image courtesy of Dr Adrian M.K. Thomas.

This was an unparalleled public response and a total of 2842 active cases of tuberculosis and 5379 cases requiring observation were discovered. The campaign was organized by the City of Glasgow, the Western Regional Hospital Board, and the Department of Health for Scotland. The campaign was well organized and a model for further campaigns. Concerns about the use of imaging in screening populations are still present today, notably with trials on the use of CT scanning in screening for lung cancer and current controversies on mammography screening for breast cancer.

References

1. **Thomas, A.M.K.** (1995). Development of diagnostic radiology. In Thomas, A.M.K., Isherwood, I., and Wells, P.N.T. (Eds), *The Invisible Light. 100 Years of Medical Radiology*, pp. 13–18. Oxford: Blackwell Science.
2. **Meadowcroft, W.H.** (1896). *The ABC of the X-Rays*. London: Simpkin, Marshall, Hamilton, Kent.
3. **Webb, S.** (1990). *From the Watching of Shadows. The Origins of Radiological Tomography*. Bristol: Adam Hilger.
4. **Banerjee, A.K.** (2000). Diagnostic imaging of the gastrointestinal tract: a historical review. *The Invisible Light*, 13, 39–46.
5. **Grainger, R.G. and Thomas, A.M.K.** (1999). History of intravascular iodinated contrast media. In Dawson, P., Cosgrove, D., and Allison, D.J. (Eds), *Textbook of Contrast Media*, pp. 3–14. Oxford: Isis Medical Media.
6. **Amdam, R.P. and Sogner, K.** (1994). *Wealth of Contrasts, Nyegaard & Co.—A Norwegian Pharmaceutical Company 1974–1985*. Oslo: Ad Notam Gyldendal.
7. **Rolfe, E.B.** (1995). History of neuroradiology. In Thomas, A.M.K., Isherwood, I., and Wells, P.N.T. (Eds), *The Invisible Light. 100 Years of Medical Radiology*, pp. 19–23. Oxford: Blackwell Science.
8. **Veiga-Pires, J.A. and Grainger, R.G.** (1982). *Pioneers in Angiography: The Portuguese School of Angiography*. Lancaster: MTP Press Ltd.
9. **Jennett, B.** (1984). *High Technology Medicine*. London: Nuffield Provincial Hospitals Trust.
10. **Harrison Orton, G. and Walsham, H.** (1906). *The Röntgen Rays in the Diagnosis of Diseases of the Chest*. London: H.K. Lewis.

Chapter 6

Computed tomographic scanning

The development of computed tomography

The impact that the EMI (Electrical and Musical Industries) or computed tomography (CT) scanner has had on investigative medicine cannot be overestimated.[1] The invention of the CT scanner marked the paradigm shift between traditional diagnostic radiology and modern medical imaging.

Within 5 years of the introduction of the CT scanner there were machines in major centres on all continents and the technique was being rapidly adopted into clinical practice. It is now difficult to imagine how medicine was practised before the introduction of CT scanning. The introduction of the CT scanner, followed by the widespread use of ultrasound and magnetic resonance imaging (MRI) has resulted in the blossoming of the radiological sciences since the 1970s. As an example, the conventional diagnosis of haemorrhage into the head following injury was difficult and uncertain. Internal injury could be inferred from a fracture of the skull or a shifted pineal gland shown on a plain radiograph or, sometimes, in neurosurgical units using ultrasound to demonstrate midline shift. Haemorrhage was also diagnosed using the invasive technique of cerebral angiography; however, doctors were obviously reluctant to perform invasive diagnostic examinations unless the chances of finding an abnormality were high. Patients with head injury were commonly admitted for neurological observations after being examined by skull radiography and were observed in hospital with a wait and see policy. Patients with significant trauma to the head now have an early CT scan under National Institute for Health and Clinical Excellence (NICE) guidelines and appropriate medical intervention can be undertaken with confidence, and many lives have been saved as a consequence. Figure 6.1 is the brochure cover for the EMI1010

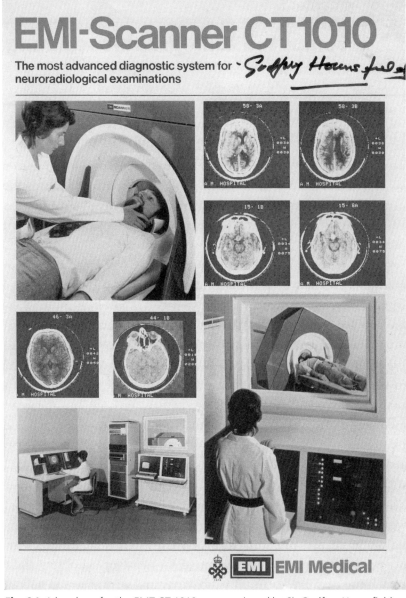

Fig. 6.1 A brochure for the EMT CT 1010 scanner signed by Sir Godfrey Hounsfield.
Included courtesy of EMI Records Limited.

scanner 'the most advanced system for neuroradiological examinations' and is signed by Godfrey Hounsfield.

The pioneer British neuroradiologist James Bull, in introducing the book of the First European Congress on Computerised Axial Tomography in Clinical Practice held in 1977, said that Hounsfield's revolutionary radiological technique was the most important advance in X-ray photography since Wilhelm Röntgen radiographed his wife Bertha's hand in November 1895 in Würzburg and that the result of Hounsfield's discovery has been to transform investigative medicine. Seldom in the history of medicine has a new discovery swept the world quite as quickly as that of CT.

Johann Radon

The history of the development of computerized axial tomography is complex and interesting.[2] Radon had published his fundamental work in 1917 on the 'Radon transform' which mathematically stated that if the line integrals of a particular property of an object, such as its density, could be known for all lines intersecting a slice of any object and coplanar with the slice, then the density can be reconstructed exactly. Allan Cormack had only become aware of the pioneering work of Johann Radon only in the late 1970s. This idea of reconstructing a function from a set of projections is important for the development of CT.

There were a number of workers who were looking at developing tomography from its earlier mechanical forms. In the 1940s Shinji Takahashi in Japan worked on the principles underlying rotational radiography and developed what we would now call sinograms. In 1957 Korenblyum and his co-workers built a medical CT scanner in Kiev in the then USSR independently of other workers. In 1960 William Oldendorf made experiments to demonstrate the feasibility of CT scanning using a rotating phantom made of nails and mounted on a rotating turntable. It is interesting to observe the number of disconnected workers considering the same problem but coming from quite different directions.

Allan Cormack and Godfrey Hounsfield

As the only nuclear physicist in Cape Town in 1955 Allan Cormack supervised the use of radioactive isotopes at Groote Schuur Hospital on a part time basis.[3] He became interested in radiotherapy treatment planning and in isodose charts. The isodose charts in use at the time assumed that the body was homogenous. Cormack realized that treatment planning could be improved if the distribution of attenuation coefficients in the body could be determined by external measurements. Cormack developed a mathematical approach to looking at the problems of variations in body tissues that are important in radiotherapy. In 1957 he performed experiments using a phantom that had circular symmetry. By 1963 Cormack was ready to make experiments on a phantom that did not have circular symmetry. The apparatus consisted of two cylinders containing a detector and a gamma ray source. The phantom lay between the two cylinders and the work was done in the summer of 1963. Cormack then considered how many measurements needed be made since only a finite number of measurements can be made with beams of a finite width. The results were presented in graphical form and were published in 1964. There was almost no response to the publication although Cormack related that the most interesting reprint request was from the Swiss Centre for Avalanche Research since the method he had described could be used for examining snow on a mountain assuming that the source or detector could be placed inside the mountain under the snow. There was certainly no commercial interest in the work of Cormack.

In the 1960s Godfrey Hounsfield was working for EMI Ltd in Middlesex.[4] Hounsfield was a remarkable man who had left school with no formal qualifications. He trained as an engineer in the Royal Air Force in the Second World War and worked on radar.[4] After the war Hounsfield worked for EMI and he built the first solid-state electronic computer in the UK. He then worked on computer memory and when that project was shelved Hounsfield investigated pattern recognition. As part of this he considered the internal structure of an object and how it could be examined. The box could be looked at from many directions using an X-ray or gamma-ray source and a radiation detector. The original apparatus was very simple and resembled that which had been used by Allan Cormack. The basis of the apparatus was a simple lathe holding the object to be examined. On opposite sides were a radiation source (initially an americium radioisotope source) and a radiation detector. The early experiments were made using Perspex phantoms of varying complexity, and the results of the transmission readings could then be analysed by the computer and presented as a series of slices in a single plane. Hounsfield developed a mathematical approach to determine the nature of the objects in the box in a process of iterative reconstruction, which he developed with Steve Bates. The iterative method of reconstruction starts with an estimated picture and the final image is built up from a series of edge readings until the final image is consistent with edge readings from each of the different angles.

Figure 6.2 is from an album made by Godfrey Hounsfield and is scanned directly from the original Polaroid photograph. It was labelled by Hounsfield as 'first picture ever' and is the first ever CT image taken by him. The readings were taken using a scintillation counter, which

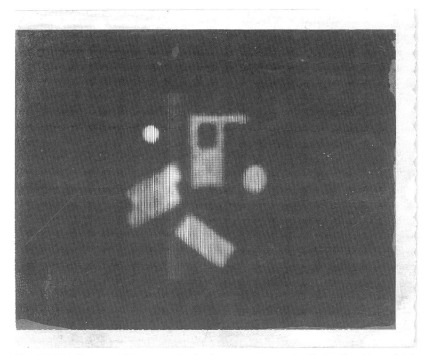

Fig. 6.2 The first ever CT scan made of a Perspex phantom by Sir Godfrey Hounsfield. Included courtesy of EMI Records Limited.

counted the gamma ray photons. It took 9 days to take the picture and 15 minutes computing time to reconstruct the picture. Following the use of Perspex phantoms a section of human brain in formalin in a Perspex box was used as a phantom. Most of the pictures from the lathe bed were scanned in 1969 and 1970.

Hounsfield now had to look for practical applications of the technique and so he approached the Department of Health and Social Security (DHSS) in London in 1968. Hounsfield met with Cliff Gregory and in October of 1968 EMI submitted a formal proposal to support the costs involved, and this project was given to Gordon Higson. In January 1969 Higson and Hounsfield with Evan Lennon, a radiologist on the staff of the DHSS, visited the EMI laboratories in Hayes. The feasibility study was completed by November 1969 and the DHSS approached three radiologists in different areas to examine the system critically. These were Frank Doyle from the Hammersmith Hospital, James Ambrose from Atkinson Morley's Hospital, and Louis Kreel from the Royal Free Hospital (who subsequently moved to Northwick Park Hospital in Harrow). There was then a period when the three radiologists worked closely with EMI. Frank Doyle supplied bone specimens, James Ambrose supplied brain specimens, and Louis Kreel supplied abdominal specimens. On 14 January 1970 there was a meeting at the DHSS to assess progress. The initial results were very promising and the group was particularly impressed that lack of definition of some specimens could be seen because of specimen deterioration. Hounsfield submitted the provisional specifications for a clinical prototype in February 1970. Because of the difficulties of abdominal scanning it was agreed that the prototype would be a brain machine and that this was to be located at Atkinson Morley's Hospital in Wimbledon, South London.

However, there were still uncertainties in the senior management at EMI who felt that the project involved considerable financial risk. There was even a suggestion that the project should be sold to an American company and careful negotiations between the DHSS and EMI were needed. An advisory team was set up in July 1970 which met regularly until August 1971. The DHSS was unsure about committing public money to more than one prototype and anticipated committing

£250,000 of public money, which was a considerable sum in those days. It was believed there would be a UK market for about 12 machines. The DHSS finally underwrote four machines, two for installation in the UK and two that EMI could sell overseas. In order to recover their money the DHSS built a royalty agreement into the EMI contract and the contract was finally signed in July 1971.

The EMI scanner

The prototype EMI brain scanner was installed in Atkinson Morley's Hospital on 1 October 1971. The neuroradiologist in charge of the unit was James Ambrose and he developed a close relationship with Godfrey Hounsfield (Figure 6.3). Ambrose is a key figure in the development of CT scanning and in modern neuroradiology.

James Ambrose had come to the UK from South Africa in 1954 to study radiology. He became interested in neuroradiology and went to work at Atkinson Morley's Hospital in 1959 where he was to spend his working life. Atkinson Morley's Hospital was in Wimbledon in South London and by 1948 it had become the busiest neurosurgical unit in London. Neurosurgery had been developed at the hospital by Wylie McKissock who had visited Stockholm and had been very impressed by the close collaboration between the surgeon Herbert Olivecrona and the radiologist Eric Lysholm. McKissock disliked the current invasive neuroradiological techniques of angiography and pneumoencephalography and James Ambrose shared his concerns. The department at Atkinson Morley's Hospital therefore actively investigated alternative imaging techniques including cranial ultrasound and nuclear medicine with the support of the physics department at St George's Hospital.

Ambrose had been working on cranial ultrasound to determining the position of the midline of the brain and so detect pathology since 1964 but the technique was uncertain and prone to artefact. Ambrose then presented his work on cranial ultrasound in 1969 to the meeting of the British Medical Association in Leicester and although the paper was well received Ambrose would admit that the technique was not generally useful. In 1969 Ambrose presented a paper at the Annual Congress

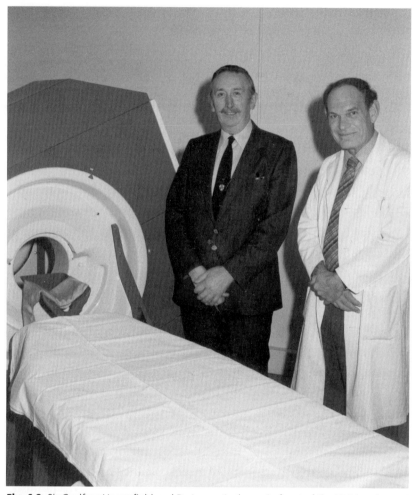

Fig. 6.3 Sir Godfrey Hounsfield and Dr James Ambrose in front of the EMI head scanner at Atkinson Morley's Hospital.

Included courtesy of EMI Records Limited.

of the British Institute of Radiology, analysing the nuclear medicine brain scans performed in 1968 at Atkinson Morley's Hospital. The hospital had performed 731 studies and although the numbers of nuclear scans were increasing, Ambrose found the number of contrast radiological studies had remained constant. Ambrose was well prepared to respond positively to Godfrey Hounsfield and to his innovative ideas regarding cranial imaging.

The prototype scanner was installed at Atkinson Morley's Hospital on 1 October 1971. It is quite remarkable that Hounsfield went from the primitive lathe bed apparatus to the prototype CT scanner in one move. This prototype CT scanner (Figure 6.4) looks very similar to modern CT scanners and currently is on display in the Science Museum in South Kensington, London. The scanning time was 4 minutes per slice with a slice thickness of a little over 1cm. A computer was not attached to the machine and the data had to be taken by car on magnetic tape to be analysed by EMI at Hayes. There was no plan at this time to have a computer attached to the scanner, and the scanner was designed to take the readings on magnetic tape for off-site processing. The data was reconstructed using an ICL 1905 mainframe computer that took 20 minutes to reconstruct a picture and an 80×80 matrix took 20 minutes. The software was written by Stephen Bates who made major contributions to early CT computing at EMI. It would have been possible to

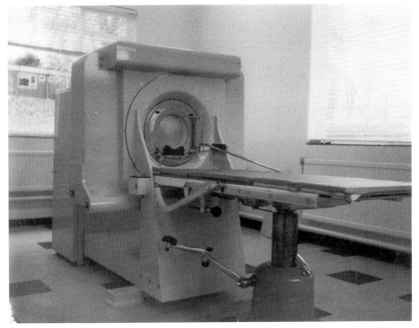

Fig. 6.4 The prototype CT scanner installed at Atkinson Morley's Hospital in South London and now at the Science Museum in South Kensington, London.

Included courtesy of EMI Records Limited.

have reconstructed the data using a 160×160 matrix but that would have taken a considerably longer time. Ambrose felt that at least 6 months of work would be needed to build up an appreciation of both the normal and the abnormal.

The first patient scanned on the new machine was a 41-year-old lady with a possible frontal lobe tumour. The data were acquired and the tapes sent to EMI with the results being returned after 2 days. The cystic tumour in the left frontal lobe was shown clearly (Figure 6.5), and Ambrose said the result caused him and Hounsfield to jump up and down like football players who had just scored a winning goal. Radiology was changed forever. The scan is presented in the opposite direction from modern scans and is viewed as a neurosurgeon would look, which is from above. Modern scans are viewed as looking from below upwards since doctors usually look up the body from below. The back of the Polaroid print has the words of Hounsfield 'original 1st PATIENT SCANNED' with his written request for it to be returned to him.

The results were presented at the Thirty-Second Annual Congress of the British Institute of Radiology that was held at Imperial College in London in April 1972. The session 'New Techniques for Diagnostic Radiology' was held on the afternoon of Thursday 20 April, and was chaired by the neuroradiologist George du Boulay. The paper presented by Ambrose and Hounsfield was called 'Computerised axial tomography (A new means of demonstrating some of the soft tissue structures of the brain without the use of contrast media)'. The paper produced a sensation with the first press announcement appearing in *The Times* on 21 April 1972. The presentation was then published as an abstract in the *British Journal of Radiology* with three papers appearing in the December 1973 issue.[1] The first paper was by Godfrey Hounsfield (from the Central Research Laboratories of EMI Limited, Hayes, Middlesex) on 'Computerised transverse axial scanning (tomography): Part 1. Description of system'. In this paper Hounsfield described and illustrated the theories behind and the applications of the new scanner. In the second paper James Ambrose (from Atkinson Morley's Hospital, London, SW10) wrote on 'Computerised transverse axial scanning (tomography):

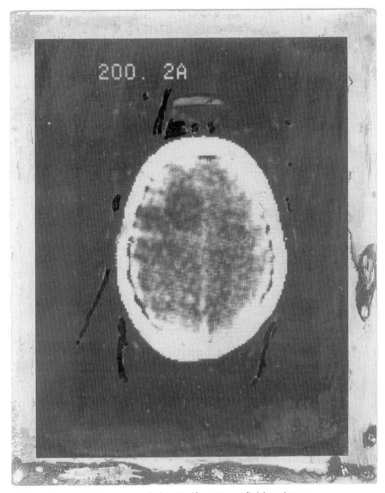

Fig. 6.5 First clinical CT scan made by Godfrey Hounsfield and team.
Included courtesy of EMI Records Limited.

Part 2. Clinical Application'. In this paper Ambrose described the technique for scanning and illustrated the scans obtained with comparisons to anatomical specimens, angiography, and nuclear medicine isotope brain scans. In the third paper B.J. Perry and C. Bridges (both from St George's Hospital in London) wrote on Computerised transverse axial scanning (tomography): Part 3. Radiation dose considerations'. This was an important topic and one that is hotly debated today.

EMI then started the production of five head scanners, one destined for the National Hospital, Queen Square, one for Manchester, one to go to Glasgow, and two for the USA, for the Mayo Clinic and for the Massachusetts General Hospital. All these machines were installed and operating by the summer of 1973. James Bull described the head scanner to the American neurologist Fred Plum. Plum estimated that USA would need at least 170 brain machines to cover the neurology and predicted that it would become unethical to practise neurology without access to the EMI scanner since it reduced the need for the currently available invasive techniques.

The Nobel Prize

The award of the Nobel Prize for Medicine or Physiology in 1979 to Godfrey Hounsfield and Allan Cormack confirmed the value of the new technique.[5] Hounsfield received many awards and was knighted by Queen Elizabeth. In 1974 James Ambrose and Godfrey Hounsfield jointly received the Barclay Prize of the British Institute of Radiology, and James Ambrose received honorary membership in 1993.

Developments in CT scanning

Whilst the new scanner was obviously clinically effective it was also very expensive and this limited its use. EMI had various problems that Melvyn Marcus outlined in the *Sunday Telegraph* of 30 July 1978 in an article entitled 'It's crisis time for scanners'. The issues that EMI had were twofold. First, there was competition from other companies and several court cases for patent infringements, including a suit filed by EMI against Ohio-Nuclear in 1976 and Pfizer in 1977. These cases involved Godfrey Hounsfield in considerable time and effort to defend. However the more significant issue was the clampdown on hospital spending in the USA under President Jimmy Carter. America was the largest market for the EMI scanner and hospitals were forced to meet very rigorous standards to justify a major or capital expenditure. However, in spite of the problems experienced by EMI and the EMI scanner, CT has continued to develop.

The expense of the CT scanner made its availability quite limited and it is only in more recent years that a CT scanner has been available in every accident unit. In the UK in the mid-1980s the CT scanner was largely restricted to regional neurological and neurosurgical units. There were many 'scanner appeals' in the 1980s led by local enthusiasts. Fund raising events were undertaken with sponsored events and the sale of items including mugs, badges, and tea towels. At Farnborough Hospital in South London a 'CAT Scanner Appeal' was made with a sponsored Land's End to John O'Groats bicycle ride. Figure 6.6 illustrates a fundraising badge from Bromley group of hospitals. The problem with these charity events was that the appeal would buy the scanner but commonly did not supply the staff, running costs, or maintenance needed. The local health district was then under an obligation to support the new scanner and replace it when necessary and radiology staff had to work harder. The positive side is that the wider availability of CT scanning emphasized the case for local provision of services. It is the availability of a CT scanner in every accident unit that has led to the transformation of clinical care.

When the team at EMI was developing the whole-body scanner it became obvious that a cross-section of the body would be of value for radiotherapy treatment planning. Before CT scanning radiotherapy

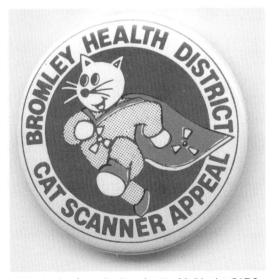

Fig. 6.6 A fundraising badge from the Bromley Health District CAT Scanner Appeal.
Image courtesy of Dr Adrian M.K. Thomas.

treatment planning was both imprecise and time consuming. There was a perceived imbalance between the accuracy of the treatment that could be delivered by the linear accelerator and the treatment plans that could be made. The CT scan enabled computer programs to guide the treatment beam with the radiotherapy planning system linked to the CT diagnostic display console. The radiation isodose distribution curves could be overlaid on the CT image and the CT density numbers (Hounsfield units) could also be used to calculate the effect of inhomogeneities in the tissues in the path of the radiation beam. Indeed, this was the very problem that Allan Cormack had been investigating in 1956. The areas to be irradiated could be defined as could the radiosensitive areas that needed to be avoided.

Many papers and presentations were made on the new technique. The British Society of Neuroradiologists met in Glasgow on 12 October 1972 and James Ambrose spoke about the new technique of computerized transverse axial scanning. In 1974 James Ambrose with Ross Paxton spoke again to the British Society of Neuroradiologists in a meeting that was held at Atkinson Morley's Hospital about his continuing experience of EMI scanning and the hospital had now scanned 650 patients. By the September of 1974 the prototype scanner had by then been installed for 2 years with the first year being devoted to evaluation; however, in the second year the machine was being put to full clinical use. James Ambrose worked with Glynn Lloyd from Moorefield's Eye Hospital to evaluate orbital disease using the 'Emiscan'. The orbits had been difficult to image using traditional techniques. The initial CT scanner used an 80×80 matrix for its image display but by 1974 a 160×160 matrix was being used and the detail obtained was improved dramatically.

The initial EMI scanner images were obtained as Polaroid photographs. The digital images could be reviewed on the scanner. By December 1974 R.A. Shields, Ian Isherwood, and R.B. Pullan from Manchester had scanned 1500 patients and were viewing the images on a console that was independent of the scanner itself.

Following the success of the head scanner, the first body scanner was installed at Northwick Park Hospital under the directorship of Louis Kreel (Figure 6.7) and by 1977 he was reviewing the results of

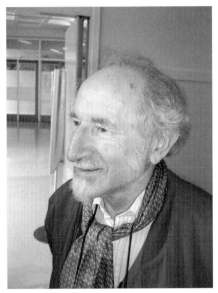

Fig. 6.7 Dr Louis Kreel, the pioneer of body CT at Northwick Park Hospital.
Image courtesy of Dr Adrian M.K. Thomas.

this EMI general-purpose scanner and investigative medicine had been transformed.

The radiation dosage to patients from the CT scanner (EMI brain and body scanners) was investigated by B.F. Watts from the National Radiological Protection Board and D.A.C. Green from EMI Medical Ltd in March 1979. They concluded that at that time dosages were similar to conventional radiography.

As the 1980s progressed, the papers describing the use of CT became increasing sophisticated and complex. Many of the techniques described at that time are now part of our routine daily practice. In the early 1980s high-resolution CT of the petrous bone was becoming commonplace and was replacing complex conventional tomography.

It should be realized that conventional techniques persisted for quite some time after the introduction of the 'Emiscan'. This was related partly to the limited availability of scanners although the scanners were still not developed fully. For example, abnormalities of the hila could often be better displayed and assessed more confidently using conventional tomography. There was also an older generation of radiologists who were well trained in the older technology and who found the introduction of new techniques problematic. It is surprising that air encephalography was still being taught on the 1981–1984 London FRCR radiology course even though the technique was long obsolete by then. The continued use of the radionuclide brain scan (RBS) in an age of CT is also interesting. It was still believed in the 1980s that as a physiological technique the RBS was complementary to the CT brain scan; however, the technique was fighting a losing battle as the number of CT scanners slowly increased. In similar manner CT was to fight a losing battle as MRI improved in quality and availability although the introduction of CT spiral volumetric scanning in the 1990s reversed the trend.

In the mid-1980s CT continued to improve in quality with technical developments including three-dimensional (3-D) imaging. The 3-D reformats were elegant and it was following the development of helical scanning that the technique came into its own.

Willi Kalender and helical scanning

Spiral CT represents a significant advance in the technology of CT scanning and has transformed and extended the clinical use of CT. The first clinical cases and performance measurements of the new technique were presented as work in progress by Willi Kalender, Peter Vock, and Wolfgang Seissler at the 75th Anniversary Meeting of the Radiological Society of North America in 1989. Thereafter the technique was fully described in a paper in *Radiology* in 1990.[6] At this time MRI was developing very rapidly and there was a question mark over the future value of CT scanning. Willi Kalender (1949–) was born in Thorr, Nordrhein-Westfalen in Germany. In 1995 he was appointed full professor and chairman of the newly established Institute of Medical Physics at the Friedrich-Alexander-University Erlangen-Nürnberg, Germany.

The development of spiral CT was made possible by the recent rapid advances in computing technology. The data acquired can now be reconstructed almost instantaneously. In spiral CT, the X-ray source rotates continuously around the patient and the table and patient simultaneously moves through the gantry holding the X-ray tube. The time for acquisition of the raw data is therefore significantly reduced and, instead of a set of individual slices through the patient, a volume is obtained. This information can be looked at in any desired plane, and as well as being displayed as a single slice the information can be presented as a 3-D image. The results that can now be obtained routinely with modern spiral CT scanners are quite amazing. We now have a greatly improved spatial resolution with virtual endoscopy and faster scanning enabling complex dynamic studies. The most dramatic improvement was made because of the provision of higher continuous X-ray power and specially designed CT X-ray tubes. The spiral scanners can image rapidly in a single held breath and have been particularly valuable in examining blood vessels and the acutely ill patient. Kalender finished his article with the words: 'Predictions are particularly difficult when they are concerned with the future'! In looking at the development of CT we have to agree with him.[7]

Multislice scanning and its clinical impact

The CT scanner has led to the modern paradigm shift in medical investigation and treatment. Traditional radiological investigation was often invasive and the resulting treatment invasive. The modern paradigm is that of non-invasive diagnosis and minimally invasive treatment. Minimally invasive treatment has at its basis an accurate pre-treatment diagnosis. The CT scanner also changes the way in which radiological images were interpreted. In traditional radiology the presence of an abnormality was commonly inferred by the distortion of normal anatomy. In the head the presence of a brain tumour could be inferred by a displaced blood vessel when filled with contrast media at angiography or from a distorted cerebral ventricle, which had been filled with air at pneumoencephalography. Both angiography and pneumoencephalography required the patient to be an inpatient and anaesthesia needed to be used since both techniques were physically unpleasant for the patient. As a contrast, the CT scan could be performed as an outpatient and the patient only had to keep still in the scanner gantry. Unlike angiography or pneumoencephalography the CT scanner showed the abnormality directly without any inference as was seen in the earlier mentioned case of the lady with the left-sided frontal lobe tumour.

This ability to see the abnormality directly has had several effects. The abnormality is shown more clearly and a likely diagnosis is easier to make and the extent of the abnormality is easier to define and so the radiological-pathological correlation is enhanced. Because the CT scan is non-invasive it can be repeated, easily unlike invasive techniques, and so the response of the disease to treatment can be assessed quite easily. This has greatly facilitated the monitoring of the effects of medical treatments in clinical trials. Since the CT scan is non-invasive the threshold for performing a radiological examination is reduced since doctors are understandably reluctant to perform potentially hazardous examinations without a very strong clinical indication. Since the introduction of the CT scanner the threshold for performing radiological investigations has reduced. While this has had the effect of considerably increasing the work of X-ray departments, it has also meant that abnormalities may be diagnosed at an earlier stage in their natural history and earlier diagnosis means treatment is facilitated. The CT scanner can be used to guide the radiologist in interventional radiology and facilitate the biopsy of tumours, the drainage of fluid collections, and radiofrequency ablation.

The development of spiral CT and now multislice scanning was made possible by advances in computing. Data no longer have to be taken away for analysis but can be reconstructed almost instantaneously. In spiral CT, the X-ray source rotation and the patient table translation are made simultaneously and so the time for acquisition of the raw data is significantly reduced. We now have improved spatial resolution with virtual endoscopy and faster scanning enabling complex dynamic studies. The most dramatic improvement was made because of the provision of higher continuous X-ray power and improvements in computers.

These new developments in CT have dramatically increased the uses of CT scanning and have replaced many conventional radiological techniques. Spiral CT with virtual endoscopy has resulted in CT colonography, which has replaced the barium enema. CT angiography can show the aorta and pulmonary vessels and the demands for CT for chest pain with aortography, pulmonary angiography, and coronary angiography have shown these vessels in elegant detail and with significant resource implications for radiology, both during the working day and also in the provision of 24/7 services in the '24-hour hospital'. Radiation exposure of the population remains a concern and modern generations of scanners use a lower dose and scan faster. CT has an increasing role in the acutely ill patient as a non-invasive accurate diagnosis is central to optimal patient care. CT is also combining with other imaging techniques in hybrid imaging and the techniques of positron emission tomography (PET)-CT and single-photon emission computed tomography (SPECT)-CT. The future of CT still remains exciting, even 40 years after its invention.

References

1. **Thomas, A.M.K., Banerjee, A.K., and Busch, U.** (2005). *Classic Papers in Modern Diagnostic Radiology*. Berlin: Springer Verlag.
2. **Webb, S.** (1990). *From the Watching of Shadows. The Origins of Radiological Tomography*. Bristol: Adam Hilger.
3. **Vaughan, C.L.** (2008). *Imaging the Elephant: A Biography of Allan MacLeod Cormack*. London: Imperial College Press.
4. **Bates, S., Beckmann, E., Thomas, A.M.K., and Waltham, R.** (2012). *Godfrey Hounsfield: Intuitive Genius of CT*. London: The British Institute of Radiology.
5. **Thomas, A.M.K.** (2012). The development of computer-assisted tomography. In Thompson G. (Ed.), *Nobel Prizes That Changed Medicine*, pp. 151–170. London: Imperial College Press.
6. **Kalender, W.A., Seissler, W., Klotz, E.,** *et al.* (1990). Spiral volumetric CT with single-breathhold technique, continuous transport, and continuous scanner rotation. *Radiology*, 176, 181–183.
7. **Kalender, W.A.** (1996). Spiral CT in the year 2000. In Rémy-Jardin, M. and Rémy, J. (Eds), *Spiral CT of the Chest*, pp. 322–329. Berlin: Springer.

Chapter 7

Magnetic resonance imaging

The study of magnetism goes back into antiquity. It was the Elizabethan physician William Gilbert who, in his treatise *De Magnete* (1600), came to the insight that the earth itself was a magnet and this accounted for the action of magnets. A globular loadstone (magnet) is a miniature of the earth and small compass needles placed near it dip in the same way that mariners' compasses are affected by the earth (Figure 7.1). Magnetism is a fundamental property of nature and is seen both in very large and very small structures.

Magnetic resonance imaging (MRI) is a relatively new radiological technique.[1,2] The development of MRI would not have been possible, however, without the mathematical principle of Fourier transformation, the discovery of which is credited to the brilliant French mathematician Jean Baptiste Joseph Fourier who served 3 years as the secretary of the Institut d'Egypte at the beginning of the nineteenth century during Napoleon's reign, and later became prefect of the Isère département in France.

Isidor Isaac Rabi (1898–1988) can perhaps be credited with the first description of the measurement of nuclear spin in his groundbreaking paper entitled 'Measurement of Nuclear Spin by the Method of Molecular Beams: The Nuclear Spin of Sodium'.[3,4] Rabi was an Austrian native who emigrated to the USA with his family and graduated in chemistry. His PhD thesis was on the magnetic properties of crystals and in 1934 he published his seminal contribution. He went on to become a professor of physics in 1937. He was able to first demonstrate and measure single states of rotation of atoms and molecules and determine the mechanical and magnetic movements of the nuclei. This was perhaps the earliest description of the principle of magnetic resonance. Rabi went on to win a Nobel Prize in Physics in 1944. Rabi was lucky and

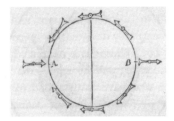

Fig. 7.1 Gilbert's terrella from *De Magnete*, 1660.

Reproduced from Silvanus P. Thompson, *Gilbert, of Colchester: An Elizabethan Magnetizer*, The Chiswick Press, London, UK Copyright © 1891.

successful, having been helped by a visit and advice from the Dutchman Cornelis Jacobus Gorter from the Netherlands in September 1937 who himself had tried similar experiments unsuccessfully.

Whereas Rabi measured the magnetic properties of nuclei it was in fact Felix Bloch and Edward Purcell (1912–1997)[5,6] who independently discovered nuclear magnetic resonance as such in 1946. Felix Bloch (1905–1983) was of Swiss origin. He eventually left Europe for the USA where he carried out his important work. In the late 1930s he carried out experiments at the Berkley cyclotron in California in which he measured magnetic movements of the neutron. Simultaneously Purcell discovered the principle of magnetic resonance working at Harvard University as a physics professor. Bloch and Purcell went on to receive the Nobel Prize in Physics in 1952. Although the fundamental physics of MRI continued to be of interest to scientists, it was a little while before the applications enabled the construction of a dedicated scanner that would enable imaging to be performed on human bodies. It is important to remember that the Russians were also working on magnetic resonance and electron spin resonance was discovered at Kazan University (in the former USSR) by Yevgeni K. Zavoisky towards the end of the war. Zavoisky had first attempted to detect nuclear magnetic resonance (NMR) in 1941 but, like Gorter, he had failed.

The pioneer Raymond Damadian (b. 1936), a physician who qualified from the Albert Einstein College of Medicine in New York, was to play a major part in the development of the MRI scanner. Having qualified as a doctor, he pursued his interest in biophysics as well as physical chemistry and mathematics and he went on to found the Fonar Corporation in 1978. He invented the MRI scanner and published a seminal paper entitled 'Tumour Detection by Nuclear Magnetic Resonance' in the journal *Science* in 1971.[7]

Other pioneers included Paul Lauterbur, who published one of the early papers on MRI in *Nature* 1973 entitled 'Image Foundation by Induced Local Interactions: Example Employing Nuclear Magnetic Resonance'. Lauterbur went on to publish over one hundred papers in the field of MRI and in 2003 Lauterbur was awarded the Nobel Prize in Physiology or Medicine along with his British colleague Peter Mansfield. Sir Peter Mansfield also can be credited with having made major contributions towards the development of the MRI scanner. A physicist by training, he worked in the University of Nottingham in the UK and contributed many of the early papers on the applications of MRI into clinical practice.[9]

Other pioneers in the early 1970s of note in magnetic resonance spectroscopy included George Radda and Rex Richards in Oxford. It was thought this application of spectroscopy would enable different characterization of tissues thus enabling more accurate clinical diagnosis to be made based not just on anatomical knowledge but also on chemical/metabolic activity.

In 1971 Raymond Damadian noted that NMR could be used to show malignant tissue in an *in vivo* animal model. After this seminal discovery several medical physicists set to work trying to build a medical scanning device using the principles of NMR. One of the earliest groups to do so was the Aberdeen group in Scotland. Professor John Mallard, professor of biomedical physics and bioengineering at the University of Aberdeen, and his team comprising Dr James Hutchison and Bill Edelstein and others set to work on this problem.

In 1974 Hutchison used an NMR image of a recently killed mouse. The pulse sequence used was in inversion recovery sequence. By 1977 Hutchison designed an air cord resistive magnet of 0.04 Tesla field strength, which was built by Oxford Instruments and became known as the body NMR machine (mark 1). In 1979 whole-body images

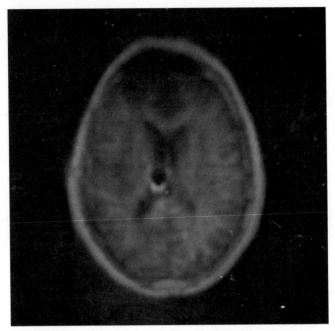

Fig. 7.2 MRI brain scan, 1980.
Reproduced with kind permission of the archive of the British Institute of Radiology.

were made but unfortunately the images were degraded by considerable movement artefact from the heart. Hutchison and his team were responsible for the spin warp technique. In 1977 the Nottingham team including Brian Worthington and Sir Peter Mansfield produced an image of a wrist using magnetic resonance. Further images were obtained of the thorax and abdomen by Ian Young and co-workers from EMI in London. They also reported the first image through the human head. Figure 7.2 shows an early head MRI from the EMI group taken in 1980. The first commercial cryogenic magnet in Europe was installed in Manchester.

By the early 1980s the clinical applications of NMR were becoming more apparent. The technique would not only image abdominal organs but could also be used in pregnancy to assess the fetus and the clinical applications in the skeletal system became more apparent.

The early MRI scanners were contained within a small copper-walled room to act as a radiofrequency shield to keep out unwanted interference. Patients were imaged on a wooden bed, which was then slid into a scanner. Today modern MRI scanners have the magnet shielded within a room that has a radiofrequency shield within the wall of the room itself.

MRI continued to develop with refinements in technique and increased field strength of the magnets. New sequences were developed to delineate disease more accurately. Pioneers from Germany, Nottingham and the Hammersmith group in the UK, and Switzerland continued to make great strides. Dennis Carr from the Hammersmith MRI group and Wolfgang Schorner from Berlin published the first images using the intravenous and MRI contrast agent gadolinium diethylenetriaminepentacetate (DTPA) dimeglumine in man. NMR spectroscopy also became a fruitful area for research resulting in two Nobel Prize winners, Richard Ernst from Switzerland in 1991 and Kurt Wüthrich in 2002 who used NMR spectroscopy for the determination of three-dimensional structures of biological molecules. Many centres contributed to the advancement of this technique including clinical applications in a whole host of areas in medicine, for example, imaging of the brain, imaging in oncology, and imaging of the musculoskeletal system. Imaging of the musculoskeletal system was completely revolutionized now that there was a technique available to look at joints more accurately than ever before without the use of radiation. Developments continued apace at the beginning of the 21st century and included open scanners for claustrophobic patients and faster scanners with greater and greater field strengths. Cardiac MRI has revolutionized cardiac imaging and even interventional procedures now are more frequently guided by MRI.

References

1. **Thomas, A.M.K., Banerjee, A.K., and Busch, U.** (2005). *Classic Papers in Modern Diagnostic Radiology*. Berlin: Springer Verlag.
2. **Isherwood, I. and Worthington, B.** (1995). Magnetic resonance imaging. In Thomas, A.M.K., Isherwood, I., and Wells, P.N.T. (Eds), *The Invisible Light. 100 Years of Medical Radiology*. Oxford: Blackwell Science.
3. **Rabi, I. and Cohen, V.W.** (1933). The nuclear spin of sodium. *Physical Review*, *43*, 582.

4. **Rabi, I. and Cohen, V.W.** (1934). Measurement of nuclear spin by the method of molecular beams: The nuclear spin of sodium. *Physical Review*, 46, 7077–7112.

5. **Bloch, F., Hansen, W.W., and Packard, M.E.** (1946). Nuclear induction. *Physical Review*, 69, 127–129.

6. **Purcell, E.M., Torrey, H.C., and Pound, R.V.** (1946). Resonance absorption by nuclear magnetic moments in a solid. *Physical Review*, 69, 37–38.

7. **Damadian, R.** (1971). Tumor detection by nuclear magnetic resonance. *Science*, 171, 1151–1153.

8. **Lauterbur, P.C.** (1973). Image foundation by induced local interactions: example employing nuclear magnetic resonance. *Nature*, 242, 190–191.

9. **Mansfield, P. and Maudsley, A.A.** (1976). Planar and line-scan spin imaging by NMR. In *Proceedings of the XIXth Congress*, pp. 247–252. Heidelberg: Ampere.

Chapter 8

Ultrasound

Ultrasound is now an integral part of medical imaging and accounts for about 40% of examinations performed in radiology departments. It has replaced many traditional radiological examinations, for example, ultrasound of the gall bladder has replaced the older oral cholecysto-gram (initially known as the Graham test).[1,2]

The physics of sound is complex and Lord Rayleigh published his *The Theory of Sound* in 1877. In 1880 Jacques and Pierre Curie described the piezoelectric effect and although there were no immediate applications this was later shown to be able to create sound waves in the sea. Following the loss of RMS *Titanic* in 1912, a British meteorologist Richardson proposed an 'Apparatus for warning a ship at sea of its nearness to large objects wholly or partly under water'[1] using sound and this was demonstrated in 1914 by the American engineer Fessenden. In the First World War, Paul Langevin, who had been a student of Pierre Curie, developed the first pie-zo-electric ultrasound transducer to detect submarines. In 1929 Sokolov proposed ultrasound for the non-destructive testing of metallic structures with the metal-flaw detector that was developed in 1940. The Second World War stimulated work on sonar (sound, navigation, and ranging) and radar (radio detection and ranging). Contact with sonar and radar was to influence many including Ian Donald and Godfrey Hounsfield.

Medical applications of ultrasound were suggested in the late 1920s. Biological effects of ultrasound were observed and as a result ultrasonic physiotherapy became popular in the 1930s and was used in the treatment of a variety of conditions, and its use continues in physiotherapy departments today.

Karl Theodor Dussik (1908–1968)

Karl Dussik was a neurologist and psychiatrist working in Vienna in the 1930s. With his younger brother Friedrich he started to investigate the use of ultrasound in medicine. Dussik was interested in neurological disease and was later in charge of the clinic for neurological disease at the Allgemeine Poliklinik (General Polyclinic) in Vienna. Ultrasound was just becoming available and was being tested as a therapeutic agent. The brothers used a through-transmission technique with two transducers, one being placed on either side of the head. They produced what they thought were echo images of the ventricles of the brain. They presented their results in 1942 and again in 1947 after the war and coined the term 'hyperphonography'. However, it was shown in 1952 that the images were artefactual and could be obtained from a dry skull in a water bath. The interpretation of any imaging technique is more difficult than might be imagined at first and this is the case in all modalities. In spite of the difficulties with the technique, the use of ultrasound to determine the position of the midline in the adult brain persisted and was being promoted in the 1970s as the Digiecho 1000 and 2000. The essential appeal of the ultrasound technique was that it might avoid the difficult neuroradiological procedures prior to computed tomography (CT) and it could also be taken to the accident unit.

However, in spite of this unpromising beginning, work on ultrasound as a diagnostic tool continued. In 1948 Douglas Howry who was training in radiology in Denver, Colorado, became interested in ultrasound and completed his first A-mode scanner in 1949. Then, working with Joseph Holmes, William Roderick Bliss, and Gerald J. Posakony, Howry constructed the first two-dimensional B-mode (or PPI, plan position indication mode) linear compound scanner, and then in 1954 the motorized 'Somascope' which was a compound circumferential scanner. The 'Somascope' was too cumbersome for clinical use. In 1952 Howry and Bliss published 'Ultrasonic visualization of soft tissue structures of the body'. Howry's major interest was in demonstrating anatomical details rather than pathology and similar to the use of X-rays 'in a manner comparable to the actual gross sectioning of structures in the pathology laboratory'.[1] The final machine, the pan scanner, was able to make compound scans of an intra-abdominal organ and the transducer rotated in a semicircular arc around the patient and this was announced in 1957.

In 1949 George Ludwig was working at the Naval Medical Research Institute at the University of Pennsylvania. Ludwig used A-mode ultrasound and examined reflected images of animal tissues. With F.W. Struthers he was able to show both gallstones and foreign bodies in tissue. These early pulse-echo A-mode ultrasound machines were developed from the metal flaw detectors.

Inge Edler and Carl Hellmuth Hertz, working in Lund in Sweden, developed the cardiac applications of ultrasound. Hellmuth Hertz was the son of the Nobel Prize Laureate Gustav Hertz. Edler was appointed director of the Laboratory for Heart Catheterization at the University Hospital of Lund in 1948 and was responsible for the preoperative diagnosis of cardiac disease. Cardiac catheterization and angiocardiography did not give sufficient information to assess the mitral valve and a correct assessment is essential before surgery. Edler considered a newer non-invasive alternative, which he thought might be like radar.

At that time Hertz was working as a graduate student at the nuclear physics department and also studied ultrasound. He was aware of the ultrasonic reflectoscope developed for non-destructive testing. Edler and Hertz borrowed a reflectoscope from the Tekniska Röntgen-Centralen, a company in Malmö that specialized in non-destructive testing, and with it they were able to obtain defined echoes moving synchronously with his heartbeat.

The pair contacted Wolfgang Gellinek of Siemens Medical in Erlangen, Germany, and borrowed a Siemens reflectoscope, receiving it in October 1953 and they started work immediately. The first cardiac ultrasound was performed in Lund in 1953 and Edler established the characteristic motion pattern obtained from the anterior leaflet of the mitral valve. He found the shape could be correlated with the severity of the stenosis. By 1955 Edler could rely on ultrasound for the diagnosis of mitral stenosis. This was the traditional M-mode echocardiography and ultrasound has become increasingly important in the examination of the heart with the introduction of two-dimensional and Doppler scanning. In 1977 Hertz and Edler received the Lasker Prize for their work.

John J. Wild (1914–2009)

John Julian Wild was born in Beckenham in South London and received his early education in London. Wild made many significant contributions to the development of medical ultrasound. From 1942 to 1944 Wild was a staff surgeon at Miller General Hospital, St Charles Hospital, and the North Middlesex Hospital in London. In 1944 he joined the Royal Army Medical Corps. Following the war he emigrated to the USA and was a Fellow in the Department of Surgery at the University of Minnesota, Minneapolis.

In 1949 Wild became interested in bowel failure. He had become interested in the treatment of blast injuries to the bowel whilst at the Miller General Hospital. In Minneapolis he wanted to find an *in vivo* technique to measure bowel wall thickness and he used ultrasound. Working with Donald Neal and using ultrasonic equipment developed during the war to train flyers to read radar maps, Wild showed that bowel wall thickness could be measured in the living. He examined a surgical specimen of stomach cancer introducing the idea of using pulse-echo ultrasound to diagnose tumours. In February 1950 he published a paper entitled 'The use of ultrasonic pulses for the measurement of biologic tissues and the detection of tissue density changes' which was received for publication on 14 November 1949. This was the first description of the use of ultrasound in cancer detection. From 1950 to 1951 he worked with Lyle French trying to diagnose cerebral tumours with ultrasound but without much success.

In 1951 Wild was examining a clinically non-malignant and a clinically malignant mass in the living, intact human breast. He actively developed the concept of non-invasive ultrasonic diagnosis and detection of cancer, particularly of the breast and the colon. In 1951 Wild and John Reid had constructed the first hospital 'echograph' on wheels. Analysis of A-mode records of breast tumours showed significant differences in the sonographic signals of neoplastic tissue when compared with normal tissue. Wild's next advance was to obtain real-time anatomical cross-sectional images of his own arm using this first self-contained small-parts scanner. He produced the first two-dimensional (B-mode) visual images in real time of the living human arm and in breast tumours, publishing the work in February 1952.

Wild and John Reid then constructed a linear B-mode machine to show tumours. This first B-mode scanner incorporated a water column that was sealed with rubber. It was the first hand-held contact scanner designed for clinical use. The scanner worked by sweeping the transducer from side to side over the breast mass. In May 1953 he produced a real-time image of a 7mm cancer of the breast. In 1954 he presented his work at the Middlesex Hospital in London where the audience included W.V. Mayneord from the Royal Marsden Hospital and it was this presentation that the young Ian Donald attended.

In 1956 Wild developed a transrectal ultrasound scanner for visualizing tumours of the colon. He also constructed a double-headed scanner for cardiac scanning. A yoke over the shoulders held transducers placed on opposite sides of the chest.

John Wild continued to work at the Medico-Technological Research Institute of Minneapolis but with private funding since earlier governmental grants had been withdrawn because of a series of legal disputes. Wild had a highly innovative approach and deservedly received the many awards he received.

Ian Donald (1910–1987)

The work of Ian Donald[3] on ultrasound transformed medical practice and at his memorial service James Willocks said, 'If you seek for his memorial, look around you. In every maternity hospital you will see ultrasound in use. A great discovery by a great man'.[3] Ian Donald was born in Liskeard, Cornwall, and following the family move to South Africa he graduated BA from the Diocesan College in Cape Town. He returned to England in 1931 and graduated in medicine at St Thomas's Hospital Medical School in 1937. During the Second World War he served as a Medical Officer in the Royal Air Force Volunteer Reserve and was mentioned in dispatches, and also was awarded the MBE for rescuing airmen from a burning aircraft. His Royal Air Force experience stimulated his interest in equipment of all kinds and he became familiar with radar and sonar. It is interesting to note that James Ambrose and Godfrey Hounsfield also served in the Royal Air Force. When he was demobilized Donald specialized in obstetrics and gynaecology. His research work at Hammersmith Hospital was in the treatment of respiratory disease in the newborn and he devised apparatus to assist neonatal respiration. Because of his passion for machines Donald was nicknamed 'Mad Donald' by some of his colleagues, who depicted him as a crazy inventor. Donald characterized himself as 'having a continuing childish interest in machines, electronic or otherwise'. His talent was appreciated by Sir Hector Hetherington and in 1954 Donald was appointed to the Regius Chair of Midwifery at the University of Glasgow.

While working in London Donald had come across the work of John Wild on the early applications of ultrasound. His became interested in the idea that sonar (Donald used the term sonar in preference to ultrasound) could be used for distinguishing solid from cystic swellings. Donald visited the Research Department of the boilermakers Babcock & Wilcox at Renfrew at the invitation of a director, who was the husband of one of his patients on whom he had performed a hysterectomy, and Donald saw their industrial flaw detector. This was an A-scope, the Kelvin Hughes Mk.4. He returned on 21 July 1955 and took with him a collection of pathological samples including fibroids and ovarian cysts that had been removed surgically in his department. He used an industrial ultrasonic metal flaw detector on these specimens and also used a large steak, which the company had supplied as a control. Donald was very encouraged by the results and visited the medical physicist W.V. Mayneord at the Royal Marsden Hospital who let Donald use his Henry Hughes Mk2B 'supersonic flaw detector'. In 1956 Thomas (Tom) Brown who worked at Kelvin & Hughes heard of Donald's interests and made contact. Tom Brown saw the problems Donald was having with the Mk2B A scanner, which supplied only one-dimensional images. Brown was able to supply Donald with a borrowed Mk 4 A-scope and a 35mm oscilloscope scanner.

In 1956 Donald and Brown were joined by John MacVicar as a Registrar in training who was later appointed Professor of Obstetrics and Gynaecology in the University of Leicester. The three of them made an intensive investigation into the value of ultrasound in differentiating between cysts, fibroids, and other abdominal tumours. The early results were disappointing and colleagues greeted the project with a mixture of scepticism and ridicule. The colleagues did have a point and looking at the early ultrasound images now the images are quite difficult to interpret. However, a dramatic case where ultrasound saved a patient's life by diagnosing a huge, easily removable, ovarian cyst in a woman who had been diagnosed as having inoperable cancer of the stomach, made people take the technique seriously. 'From this point', Ian Donald wrote, 'there could be no turning back'.[3] The trio of Ian Donald, John MacVicar, and Tom Brown eventually appeared in print in *The Lancet* of 7 June 1958 under the somewhat arid title 'Investigation of Abdominal Masses by Pulsed Ultrasound'.[1] This paper is probably the most important paper on medical diagnostic ultrasound ever published. In eight pages it described the experience of 100 patients with 12 illustrations of B-mode sonograms of the gravid uterus, ovarian cysts, fibroids, ascites, and normal and pathological conditions. The prototype B-mode scanner gantry was depicted and the probe and the Mark 4 flaw detector with which images were made. The safety of diagnostic ultrasound was also discussed and this was to be a continuing concern to Donald.

In 1959 Ian Donald had determined that echoes could be obtained from the fetal head, and his group used head measurement to assess fetal size and growth. The new Queen Mother's Hospital opened in Glasgow in 1964 and fetal cephalometry became the standard method to assess intrauterine growth. By 1961 Donald saw the sonar as ancillary to radiology and he speculated on what might be achieved in time in the hands of radiologists were they to embrace the technique.[4] There was a comprehensive ultrasonic diagnostic department installed alongside the Department of Radiology at the Queen Mother's Hospital in Glasgow.

Early ultrasound was technically demanding and very dependent on the operator. The ultrasound beam had to be perpendicular to the interface for an echo to return to the probe (Figure 8.1[4]). A compound scan could be made by overlapping a series of sector scans (Figure 8.2[4]).

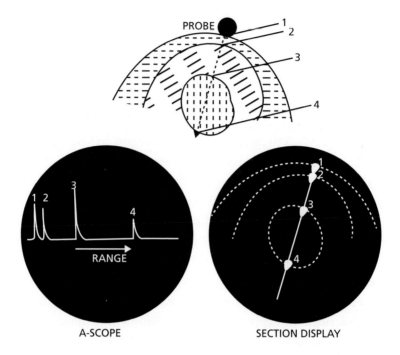

Diagram showing how interfaces at 2, 3 and 4, are represented by A-scope (left) and cross- sectional display (right)

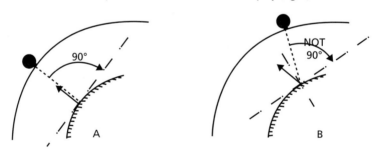

Ultrasonic beam must be perpendicular to interface (as at A) for echo to return to probe.

Fig. 8.1 Technique of ultrasound from Ian Donald and Tom Brown, 1961.

Reproduced with permission from Donald I and Brown TG, Demonstration of Tissue Interfaces within the body by Ultrasonic Echo Sounding, *British Journal of Radiology*, Vol. *34*, No. 405, pp. 539–546, Copyright © 1961 British Institute of Radiology, DOI: 10.1259/0007-1285-34-405-539.

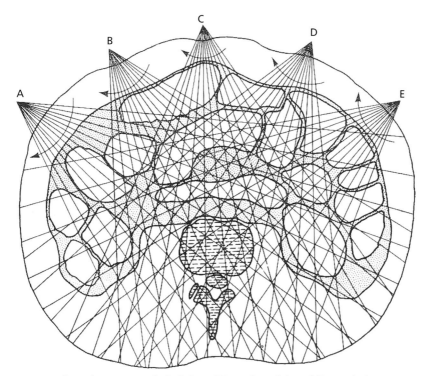

Scanning pattern. A, B, C, D and E are the origins of five typical overlapping sector scans, each of which has a mean direction towards the centre of the cross-section. In practice, a sector scan is made every 5° or so around the skin, so that each tissue interface is scanned from a large number of different angles

Fig. 8.2 Principle of compound sector scanning demonstrated by Ian Donald, 1961.

Reproduced with permission from Donald I and Brown TG, Demonstration of Tissue Interfaces within the body by Ultrasonic Echo Sounding, *British Journal of Radiology*, Vol. *34*, No. 405, pp. 539–546, Copyright © 1961 British Institute of Radiology, DOI: 10.1259/0007-1285-34-405-539.

The early images are difficult to interpret even with the benefit of labelled images (Figure 8.3[4]).

However, by 1966 Donald was to complain that the workload was beginning to rise at a rate that threatened to become unmanageable, somewhat echoing the sentiments of John McIntyre at the Electrical Pavilion many decades earlier. Donald said 'no less than 28% had undergone ultrasonic examination at some time in pregnancy'.[3] Donald also said 'A plea is made for sonar being accepted as an ancillary diagnostic

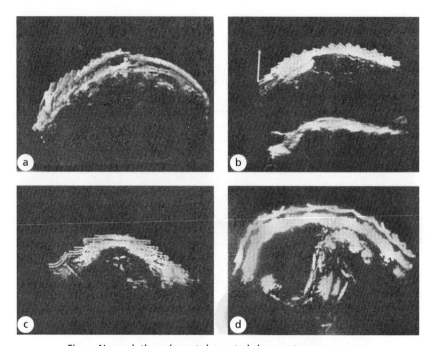

Fig. a. Normal, though protuberant abdomen; transverse scan;
bowel echoes prevent deeper penetration
Fig. b. Huge pseudomucinous ovarian cyst in longitudinal section
Fig. c. Two sets of foetal echoes. Twins at 10½ weeks gestation
Fig. d. Ovarian cyst and pregnant uterus in transverse section

Fig. 8.3 Abdominal scans by Ian Donald, 1961.

Reproduced with permission from Donald I and Brown TG, Demonstration of Tissue Interfaces within the body by Ultrasonic Echo Sounding, *British Journal of Radiology*, Vol. *34*, No. 405, pp. 539–546, Copyright © 1961 British Institute of Radiology, DOI: 10.1259/0007-1285-34-405-539.

technique by the radiological world already accustomed to visual diagnostic techniques'.[3] By 1969 ultrasound techniques were established but it took many years for radiologists to embrace the technique fully. The attitude of radiologists is now difficult to understand when the importance of ultrasound in radiology departments is obvious. Donald was to return to the theme in 1975 in his Mackenzie Davidson Memorial Lecture when he said:

> Sonar indeed employs a different energy spectrum from that of Roentgenology and the information yield is consequently different but the whole ever-increasing science and art of existing visual diagnostic techniques can now embrace new

horizons by adopting sonar not as a rival but as a complementary discipline. Whether the world of radiology likes it or not it will assuredly come to recognize and meet the challenge in the future.[5]

Writing in the 1969 edition of his classic textbook *Practical Obstetric Problems*[6] Donald described the value of sonar for studying the first-trimester fetus, observing fetal growth, estimating fetal maturity, locating the placenta, the safe and early diagnosis of twins, differential diagnosis of 'large for dates', bleeding in early pregnancy, diagnosing fetal death, diagnosis of hydatidiform mole, and not as an alternative but as an adjunct to radiography. He did not include the assessment of fetal anomalies, which was to develop as ultrasound machines improved. Throughout his career Donald was concerned with ethical and moral issues in gynaecology and obstetrics—and ethical issues are so important today. Ultrasound raises many ethical issues including antenatal screening for fetal anomalies and fetal sex determination, and the selective termination of pregnancy. Ian Donald died in 1987 and is buried in the Essex village of Paglesham.

Doppler ultrasound

In 1842 Christian Johann Doppler (1803–1853) described the effect named after him, the apparent difference in pitch when a source of waves (whether in the sound, the light, or the radiofrequency spectrum, or other spectrum) is moving towards or away from the observer. The Doppler effect has many applications including radar, navigation, astronomy, and medical ultrasound.

In 1955 the Japanese physicist Shigeo Satomura (1919–1960) began using microwave and ultrasound in industrial research. Kinjiro Okabe, his supervisor, suggested Satomura apply his ultrasound techniques to medical diagnosis. In collaboration with the cardiologists T. Yoshida and Yasaharu Nimura from Osaka University Hospital, they made measurements of the heart and looked at pulsation of the peripheral and eye blood vessels. In December 1955, Satomura published his first paper entitled 'A new method of the mechanical vibration measurement and its application', and he showed that Doppler signals can be obtained from the moving heart when scanned with 3MHz ultrasonic waves. Together with Ziro Kaneko, they made a Doppler flowmeter to measure the Doppler signal from these vessels. These works were part of Satomura's thesis, which he presented in November 1959. From July 1958 Satomura and his group started studying the extracranial cerebral blood supply using the Doppler flowmeter and pioneered early transcutaneous flow analysis of the carotid vessels in health and vascular disease. Sadly in 1960 Shigeo Satomura died at the early age of 41 of a subarachnoid haemorrhage.

Doppler applications in ultrasound continued to develop with the introduction of spectral analysis. In the late 1980s colour Doppler was introduced. The advantage of Doppler as applied to ultrasound is that it provides physiological information as well as anatomical detail. Major applications of Doppler ultrasound now include cardiac, carotid, and peripheral vascular imaging.

The development of ultrasound

Ultrasound has continued to develop from these early pioneers and what now seems such primitive apparatus. In 1968 Stuart Campbell described both the A- and B-mode scans to measure the fetal biparictal diameter and his technique became the standard for the next 10 years. The early images used bi-stable cathode ray tubes with a low dynamic range but failed to give information on echo amplitude. The development of grey scaling needed to expand both the diagnostic capability and accuracy of a B-scan. Early images were recorded on videotape, film, and thermal printers. The early dedicated scanners were compound B-scanners with the probe held on a gantry being moved across the patient in a series of overlapping arcs with the image gradually built up (Figure 8.2). The advantage of this type of scanner is that it could show larger abnormalities and the field of view of the early real time scanners was limited. In 1964 multielement linear electronic arrays were described by Werner Buschmann.

The major revolution in diagnostic ultrasound was the development of the real-time scanner which changed the practice of ultrasound. The Siemens 'Vidoson' used three individual rotating transducers housed in front of a parabolic mirror with a water coupling system and produced

15 images every second. In 1968 Hofmann and Holländer described 'Intrauterine diagnosis of hydrops fetus universalis using ultrasound' and this is probably the first description of a fetal malformation using ultrasound. In 1969 Malte Hinselmann, using the Vidoson, showed fetal cardiac pulsation from 12 weeks of gestation. The Vidoson was a popular machine particularly in continental Europe. The early ultrasound machines were of low resolution when compared with modern apparatus and even in 1970 neither ultrasound nor nuclear medicine could distinguish between obstructive and intrahepatic causes of jaundice. Techniques and apparatus slowly improved and by 1972 the Danish ultrasound pioneer Hans Holm was writing on errors and pitfalls in abdominal ultrasound and by November 1972 he and his group had scanned more than 4000 abdomens. Hans Holm was a pioneer in the use of ultrasound for intervention including biopsy and drainage that now constitute a large component of ultrasound work.

In 1971 Ellis Barnett and Patricia Morley from the Western Infirmary in Glasgow described urinary tract space-occupying lesions using a prototype version of the Nuclear Enterprises Diasonograph with compound B-scan images before the development of the grey scale. By the mid-1970s the grey-scale technique made ultrasound considerably easier, including for placental location. By the end of the decade ultrasound had improved with the diagnosis of jaundice and pancreatic disease becoming much easier but now ultrasound had to compete with early CT. Also by the end of the 1970s transrectal ultrasound of the prostate was being performed with the radial scanner incorporated into a special chair.

The scope of ultrasound increased gradually and was having profound effects on clinical practice and in particular its use in the complications of early pregnancy revolutionized the care of pregnancy. The mechanical sector scanner was a real advance on previous ultrasound machines and some companies produced a single machine incorporating a mechanical sector scanner with a compound B-scanner. Ultrasound was increasingly used in pregnancy as the 1980s progressed and Pat Farrant from Northwick Park Hospital described the early ultrasound diagnosis of fetal bladder neck obstruction, and in 1981 with Hylton Meire she published a study establishing the normal fetal limb lengths in pregnancy. As the 1980s progressed there was increasing use of imaging-guided biopsy procedures including real-time biopsy of liver lesions using a needle inserted into the central canal of a real-time linear-array ultrasound probe. By the mid-1980s ultrasound guidance using a spring loaded handle containing a Tru-Cut® type core biopsy needle was being performed.

The question of who undertakes ultrasound is interesting. In many countries ultrasound is performed only by physicians. In 1992 the group including Isobel Shirley, Fiona Bottomley, and V.P. Robinson from Hillingdon Hospital in Uxbridge, led by Shirley, was reporting on routine radiographer screening for fetal abnormalities in an unselected low-risk population. This is of interest for several reasons. The screening was undertaken by radiographers (now called sonographers) and not by doctors, and the population was of low risk. There are considerable ethical implications related to antenatal screening. Routine antenatal ultrasound is now a routine part of pregnancy in the UK and in many other countries. The group at Hillingdon Hospital had been offering routine ultrasound screening since July 1986.

Three-dimensional (3-D) ultrasound was introduced in 1984 by Kazunori Baba from the University of Tokyo, Japan, with the creation of 3-D fetal images in 1986. The 3-D images depend on complex computing. Three-dimensional scanning can show information not revealed by conventional scanning but as a technique it has not been widely taken up for routine clinical use. There are, however, companies who provide 3-D fetal facial scans as a 'bonding' scan separate from a clinical use. There are obvious ethical issues in the use of medical imaging for social indications.

FAST ultrasound and bedside ultrasound

As the decades have passed, ultrasound machines have become ever more compact and portable. These small high-quality machines can be used at the bedside and in the emergency room. Many procedures that were traditionally performed blind are now undertaken with confidence under ultrasound guidance in a clinical environment.

These procedures include the placement of chest drains and central venous lines. Ultrasound training is now part of the training of junior chest physicians and anaesthetists. In the acute setting FAST (focused abdominal sonography in trauma) is used in the initial assessment of chest and abdominal pathology. Modern ultrasound machines are small and portable and there are now ultrasound machines that are the size of a smartphone. Given the pace of ultrasound development, further significant improvements seem certain.

References

1. **Thomas, A.M.K., Banerjee, A.K., and Busch, U.** (2005). *Classic Papers in Modern Diagnostic Radiology*. Berlin: Springer Verlag.
2. **Fleming, J.E.E.** (1995). 'Inaudible sound'—medical ultrasound. In Thomas, A.M.K., Isherwood, I., and Wells, P.N.T. (Eds), *The Invisible Light: 100 Years of Medical Radiology*, pp. 71–74. Oxford: Blackwell Science.
3. **Willocks, J. and Barr, W.** (2004). *Ian Donald. A Memoir*. London: RCOG Press.
4. **Donald, I. and Brown, T.G.** (1961). Demonstration of tissue interfaces within the body by ultrasonic echo sounding. *British Journal of Radiology*, 34, 539–546.
5. **Donald, I.** (1961). New diagnostic horizons with sonar. *British Journal of Radiology*, 49, 306–315.
6. **Donald I.** (1969). *Practical Obstetric Problems*. London: Lloyd Luke.

Chapter 9

Digital imaging, picture archiving, and communication systems

The development of digital processing

Digital radiography has completely transformed medical imaging.[1] The traditional film stores are a thing of the past (Figure 9.1). The digital images may be stored electronically like this 'hand with ring' radiographed on 8 November 2005, exactly 110 years after Röntgen's discovery (Figure 9.2).

The first radiographic images were recorded directly on to photographic media. This started to change starting in the early 1930s when Helga Christensen developed an optical device with which images from the fluorescent screen could be photographed directly on to 25mm roll film. In the 1940s, A. Bowers from Oude Delft Enterprises in the Netherlands developed a 40cm input screen and recorded on to 70mm roll film. Robert Janker in Germany used this camera to record images in rapid succession and avoided the previously needed rapid cassette changes.

The first image-intensifier was developed by J.W. Coltman from Westinghouse in 1948. This image intensifier used an electron-optical design and by 1953 it was put into clinical use. The early image intensifier systems were viewed directly using a mirror but developments in the television camera which could scan the output of the image intensifier allowed for the development of complete X-ray-television systems. Fenner, working for Siemens, reported on the characteristic values of image intensifiers in 1967 and the use of electron-optical image intensifiers in radiological diagnostics.

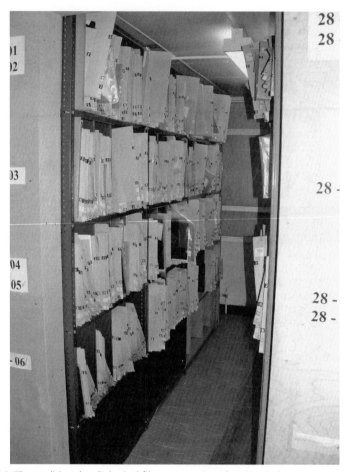

Fig. 9.1 The traditional radiological film store at Bromley Hospital.
Image courtesy of Dr Adrian M.K. Thomas.

Another major advance was the use of a caesium iodide input screen instead of the usual zinc cadmium sulphide input, and this resulted in brighter and better defined images with higher contrast. The immediate effect of the image intensifier was that fluoroscopy was now performed in a lit room and the need for dark adaptation with the use of red goggles for fluoroscopy in a dark room was abolished. As a result it was easier to perform procedures since the radiologists, radiographers, and nurses could now see clearly what they were doing. So, for example, Melvin Judkins from Portland, Oregon, and F. Mason Sones from

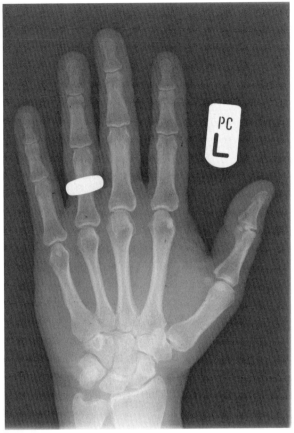

Fig. 9.2 A hand with a ring, a computed radiograph from 8 November 2005, 110 years after the discovery of X-rays.

Image courtesy of Dr Adrian M.K. Thomas.

Cleveland, Ohio, became the first to use this new image intensifier technique successfully for coronary angiography.

Towards the end of the 1970s early work in digital subtraction angiography (DSA) was undertaken by Heintzen (1976) in Kiel, Nudelman (1977) in Arizona, and Mistretta (1978) in Wisconsin. In the1980s analogue to digital converters and electronic computing systems were adapted to the conventional fluoroscopic image intensifiers and television systems resulting in further advances in digital techniques. In 1980 Philips introduced the first digital subtraction angiography system, digital vascular imaging, which ushered in the digital age of conventional radiology. It made use of the image intensifier and television technique and converted the analogue signal into digital format. Several DSA systems appeared in the mid-1980s including a unit at Lewisham Hospital in South London. The results were dramatic and were enhanced by the new generation of non-ionic contrast media that were coming into clinical use. As a result the patient was able to keep still during angiography and the digital images were available immediately without the need for darkroom processing as was needed with angiography using the traditional AOT or Puck changers. In 1986 Siemens improved the image matrix standard from 512×512 to 1024×1024. The initial results in angiocardiography with the HICOM digital system in 1990 showed an image quality that was similar to cine film. Intravenous DSA has now been superseded by computed tomography (CT) and magnetic resonance angiography.

Digital radiography for plain films developed quite slowly compared with CT and fluoroscopy. The conversion of X-ray energy patterns into digital signals using scanning laser-stimulated luminescence opened the door to new techniques in digital radiography. The basic principles were developed in 1983 by H. Kato and others at Fuji Film in Japan in 1983. An early unit for digital chest radiography was developed by G.T. Barnes and others at the University of Alabama in cooperation with Picker International. In 1982 to 1983, in the first clinical field study, 400 patients were examined over a 6-month period. The Philips Thoravision of 1994 was the first digital chest radiography unit using a selenium detector.

Accompanying the advances being made at the start of the digital information age, ideas were developed to build up a complete digital diagnostic system for radiography and fluoroscopy. In 1995, Lee, Cheung, and Jeromin patented a new digital detector for projection radiography that incorporated a multilayer structure that included a thin-film detector array, a selenium X-ray semiconductor, a dielectric layer, and a top electrode. This prototype digital radiography technology electronically converted the X-ray photons into a digital image. Digital radiography involves a direct capture of images in a digital format that can be sent to a variety of display devices and to storage. This new technology enabled conventional radiographic imaging to change from a film-based system to an effective digital system.

In 1997, John Rowlands and others from Toronto, Canada, described a projection real-time detector for dynamic X-ray imaging, thereby replacing the conventional X-ray image intensifier with an active matrix flat panel device. This digital radiography and fluoroscopy is now replacing conventional X-ray detector technologies and hospitals are moving to digital systems. A picture archiving and communication system (PACS) is linked to a RIS (radiology information system) and then to a hospital-wide electronic patient record. Radiological studies can now be image linked to other healthcare providers and the old hard copy is now only a memory. The sheer volume of data that is generated by modern medical imaging is a significant proportion of the data flow in any healthcare facility and the information technology (IT) needs to be robust with the increasing clinical dependence on radiology.

Teleradiology

The first use of teleradiology was probably in 1959 when Dr Alberta Jutra linked two hospitals in Montreal. The hospitals were five miles apart and Jutra used a coaxial cable to share videotaped fluoroscopic studies. Jutra was very perceptive and suggested that a network connection from hospitals to doctor's offices facilitated the exchange of radiological information and emphasized the need 'to determine the efficiency, usefulness and economy of roentegenologic teleconmmunication.'[1] There were a series of studies of teleradiology in the 1980s in the USA, with a large field trial in 1982 located at the Malcolm Grow Hospital in Andrews Air Force Base which served as a central location providing radiographic interpretation to one civilian and three military clinics. The radiographs were scanned using a video camera with a freeze frame constructing a $512\times512\times8$-bit matrix. The digitized X-ray images from the remote clinic were sent via telephone lines to the central medical centre and the radiological report was returned again by telephone lines. The results of the trial were successful and in 1984 the Uniformed Services University in Bethesda, Maryland replaced Malcolm Grow Hospital as the hub linking the four sites. In the 1984 study a matrix density of 1024×1024 pixels was used. The radiographs were scanned and converted to a digitized image. The results of the 1982 and 1984 trials were very encouraging with only a few discrepancies between the video and film reports. Lewis Carey reviewed teleradiology in 1985 and predicted that improved access to radiologists, for 24 hours each day, would lead to a level of service that was 'heretofore not possible.'[1]

This has proven to be the case and studies are now routinely reported by radiologists at home or transmitted between hospital sites for reporting. Images may be reported in another country; however, there are clinical and legal concerns. Nevertheless, technology continues to advance apace and it is now possible for radiological images to be reviewed on a tablet computer.

PACS and HIS/RIS

In 1971, at the European Congress of Radiology in Amsterdam, there was a symposium on the applications of computers in diagnostic radiology. Following this there were a series of meetings throughout the 1970s and towards the end of the decade the concept of digital image communication and digital radiology was introduced. With the support of the International Society of Optical Engineering the first conference and workshop on 'Picture Archiving and Communication Systems (PACS) for Medical Applications' was held in January 1982. In 1979, Heinz Lemke from the Technical University of Berlin had published the earliest paper that proposed the concept of PACS.

PACS as an idea incorporates multimedia electronic medical record, medical diagnostic workstations, and local and global IT network communications. However, there were major cost considerations which were the main reason why PACS was not started before the mid-1980s. The first clinical paper was published by J.A. Parker and others from the Nuclear Medicine Department at Beth Israel Hospital in Harvard Medical School. PACS was implemented for digital nuclear medicine images and was integrated with a radiology reporting system and gamma cameras. The advantage of starting with nuclear medicine was the relatively lower requirement for display, communication, and storage when compared with other radiological modalities. Nuclear medicine was also the first radiological modality that used computers for functional analysis.

Certain design principles used in the early PACS have remained reasonably constant. The use of standard off-the-shelf hardware and software offered the opportunity to communicate with a wide range of nuclear medicine cameras from different manufacturers and to be able to display and analyse data from all of them. Insisting on three levels of backup and redundancy results in a concept of a mini-PACS design, where each section of a radiology department has its own stand alone PACS. This was the model chosen at Farnborough Hospital in South London where a mini-PACS was started in the ultrasound department and then gradually rolled out to the rest of the department when its value had been proven.

In the UK the first attempt to create a fully filmless radiology department was at St Mary's Hospital at Paddington, London. Oscar Craig had met with Harald Glass, the Regional Scientific Officer, on 11 March 1982. Funding was requested from the Department of Health and Social Services. In June 1985 the Minister of Health promised funding and in November of that year a paper entitled 'Diagnostic Radiology Without films' was published in *The Practitioner* describing this new concept. However, it became apparent that the technology in 1985 was not adequate for the enormous task proposed. There was no filmless X-ray cassette, no clear means to rapidly transmit the vast amount of data, and little knowledge about the role of image compression. The images were not acceptable for the primary diagnosis of plain film abnormalities. In 1987 Oscar Craig gave a talk at Hammersmith Hospital and David Alison became interested in developing an entirely filmless hospital. This was proposed in the late 1980s and coincided with current technological developments. The British government gave a grant in 1990, computed radiography was introduced in 1993, and Hammersmith Hospital became filmless in 1996.

Developments were also taking place in other hospitals in Europe. In the Netherlands, Dr Bakker and others worked on 'The Dutch PACS Project'. This was sponsored by the Ministry of Health Care and based at

Utrecht University Hospital and was carried out between 1986 and 1989 with the aim of evaluating a Philips PACS prototype and to research the relationship between PACS and hospital information systems (HIS), the quality of diagnostic images, and an assessment of the technology. The first 'digital reading room' was built at Utrecht University Hospital with the first coupling of PACS–RIS. They accomplished the complete digitization of a small medical intensive care unit and the images and reports could be accessed at all times. The referring clinicians were very enthusiastic about the project since the radiological images were easily accessed without delay. The HIS and PACS were linked and the reports could be viewed on the PACS workstation. It was concluded that earlier availability of radiological images would increase the speed of diagnosis and treatment which would reduce the average length of inpatient stay. At that time it was concluded that a PACS at Utrecht University Hospital would be approximately four times as expensive as conventional radiography although it was estimated that by the year 2000 the cost of PACS would be the same as that of a conventional film-based system.

One of the few multivendor PACS installations began in 1986 at the University Hospital of Brussels working with the Multidisciplinary Research Institute for Medical Imaging Science. The University of Brussels was concerned about communication in hospitals and particularly communication between systems and also between users and systems. Working with others they were concerned with modelling the PACS–HIS coupling, evaluating image transfer using high-speed networks, developing network structures, developing a multimedia software database that would enable intelligent information retrieval, and designing an adaptive user interface to increase diagnostic efficiency.

The first PACS project in Austria started in 1985 as a project between Siemens and the Department of Radiology in the University Hospital of Graz. The Department of Radiology at Graz had developed an in-house RIS and they contacted Siemens in 1985 to initiate a PACS pilot project. The aim of this PACS–RIS was for a sequential implementation that would meet the needs of both radiologists and clinicians. There would be digital acquisition, storage and communication of radiological images from all imaging modalities, and gradual introduction of softcopy reporting and filmless working. The group in Graz were probably the first in Europe to produce an operational PACS–RIS coupling. This culminated at the end of the 1980s in the new Danube Hospital in Vienna which was filmless and fully digital. It was led by Walter Hruby who was the head of the Radiology Department and who worked in cooperation with Siemens.[2] The installation began in 1991, and it was shown that the costs of digital radiography were no greater than in a conventional department.

The changes in computing technology and its influence on radiology has been astonishing with an evolutionary revolution or as Water Hruby puts it, a digital (r)evolution in radiology. It has developed from a fruitful cooperation between radiology departments, industry, and government ministries. No one group could do it alone. PACS is no longer confined to academic departments but is spreading to many hospitals and is profoundly changing all aspects of how we work. PACS gives us fast and reliable access to radiology and speeds up reporting, saves time, produces a better diagnosis, and results in an improvement in the quality of healthcare. Our film stores and cabinets of paper reports are now but a receding memory.

References

1. **Carey, L.S.** (1985). Teleradiology: part of a comprehensive telehealth system. *Radiologic Clinics of North America*, 23(2), 357–362.
2. **Thomas, A.M.K., Banerjee, A.K., Busch, U.** (2005). *Classic Papers in Modern Diagnostic Radiology*. Berlin: Springer Verlag.

Chapter 10

Interventional radiology

The term interventional radiology was not actually coined until 1967 by Alexander Margulis, the distinguished American gastrointestinal radiologist, who used the term to describe the growing body of manipulative procedures performed by physicians skilful in radiological techniques and experienced in the clinical problems.[1] Since the dawn of radiology over 100 years ago physicians realized that imaging techniques could potentially be used to guide both diagnostic and therapeutic procedures for the benefit of patients. The earliest descriptions go back to the 1920s when interventional radiology was first used to treat intussusception in children. The first radiological puncture of a gallbladder both in cadavers and in man was reported as early ago as 1921 by Burkhart and Müller in a German surgical journal.[2]

Development of angiography

Early experiments on angiography were soon carried out after the discovery of X-rays. People quickly realized that postmortem anatomy could be studied with X-rays following the injection of blood vessels with opaque substances. One of the earliest of such experimenters was Franz Exner, who apparently injected the hand of a cadaver with Teichmann's mixture (lime cinnabar and petroleum). This was injected via the brachial artery. The results were presented at the Chemical Physical Society of Vienna on 18 January 1896. A follow-up experiment by the physicists Haschek and Lindethal in Vienna is often considered the first arteriogram.[3] In the UK, N. Raw from Manchester published a skiagram of the artery in *The Lancet* in December 1896. In 1899 at St Thomas's Hospital an arteriogram was performed of a dead infant and published in the *Archives of the Roentgen Ray*. These were perhaps the first earliest demonstrations of the arterial system in man. Sicard and Forrestier are perhaps credited with performing the first angiography in humans when they injected Lipiodol droplets into the antecubital vein followed then by the journey into the pulmonary vessels. Berberich and Hirsch introduced strontium bromide and in 1924 Brookes used sodium iodide for femoral arteriography with reasonable results and good demonstration of the vascular anatomy. In the 1920s sodium iodide was the preferred contrast medium for angiography.

Cerebral angiography was pioneered by Moniz from Portugal.[4] Moniz was to go on to win a Nobel Prize in Physiology or Medicine and was a distinguished neurosurgeon and writer. Dos Santos conducted studies on abdominal arteriography in the 1920s and pioneered translumbar abdominal aortography which was still being performed in the 1980s (Figure 10.1). Cardiac angiography was pioneered by Forssmann who passed a catheter from the antecubital vein to his heart and went on to image the catheter within his heart and demonstrated the right heart and the pulmonary circulation with this new technique. Angiography in the early days in the 1930s and 1940s involved surgical exploration followed by injection. Serial catheterization was reported by Ichikawa, Farinas, and also by Radner in Lund, Sweden. Radner in 1947 introduced arterial catheterization from the radial artery following surgical dissection and developed arch aortography.

In the 1950s percutaneous arteriography were conducted more frequently by doctors following the invention of the Seldinger technique for passing catheters. Improvements in guidewire technology by coating them with Teflon to prevent clots occurred in the 1960s. This was a decade of marked advancement in the field of angiography. Digital subtraction angiography was initiated by Mistretta and his colleagues in Madison, USA, and also by Heintzen and workers in Kiel in Germany. This was a popular technique in the 1980s and early 1990s. Pioneering names in the field of angiography include Amplatz who devised several catheters. Abrahams also made major contributions in the field of angiography and was notable for producing some of the early text books in this field one of which has been regarded as the bible of angiographers.

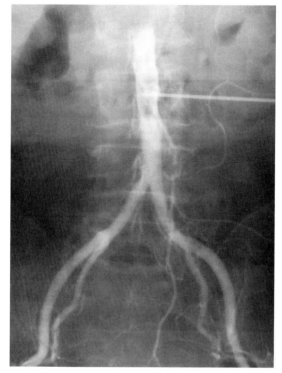

Fig. 10.1 A trans-lumbar aortogram from 1983.

Image courtesy of Dr Adrian M.K. Thomas.

Werner Forssmann (1904–1979)

Perhaps the best-known pioneer in the field of interventional radiology and angiography is Dr Werner Forssmann, a physician from a small town in Germany called Eberswalde who in 1929 performed the first human cardiac catheterization. Forssmann was a maverick as often is the case with great pioneers. He was a self-experimenter and is claimed to have catheterized himself. This did not please his bosses and he was sacked and had to switch from a career in cardiology to a career in urology. Forssmann, however, although having met initial hostility to his pioneering techniques, was rewarded with a Nobel Prize in Physiology or Medicine 1956 for his contribution to cardiac catheterization. It was in 1941 that Cournand and Richards employed cardiac catheterization as a diagnostic tool and measured cardiac output and they were also awarded the Nobel Prize in 1956 along with Forssmann for their contributions to the pioneering procedure of cardiac catheterization, a procedure which has now become routine and commonplace and is the bread and butter of cardiological interventional work.

Another great pioneer in this field was a Dr F. Mason Sones who made great pioneering strides in the fluoroscopic study of congenital heart defects. He inadvertently injected contrast medium into coronary arteries in 1959 and performed the first coronary angiogram.[5] He was a great advocate of the brachial artery approach for coronary angiography and went on to win an Albert Lasker award in 1983 for his contribution to medical science. F. Mason Sones spent most of his working life at the Cleveland Clinic in Ohio, USA, which became a world centre for cardiology.

Seldinger and his technique

Today the name of Seldinger is almost synonymous with catheterization. He was born in Mora in Sweden in 1921 and trained in medicine at the Karolinska Institute. He is credited with describing the process of percutaneous arteriography and percutaneous puncture of vessels which is still used today more than 50 years after its discovery. His pioneering paper was entitled 'Catheter Replacement of the Needle in Percutaneous Angiography' and was published in 1953 in the journal *Acta Radiologica*.[6] His technique enabled the development of superselective catheterization of vessels and embolization as well as enabling applications in non-vascular areas such as catheter drainage of abscesses. The great interventional radiologist Herbert Abrahams wrote about Seldinger's contribution mentioning that 'in the movement of angiography from the part of a bit player to that of a protagonist in a scenario of diagnostic medicine no single contribution has weighed more heavily than the technique developed by Seldinger'.[6] Seldinger's original description was not met with great enthusiasm by his chief of radiology at the Karolinska Institute though. In fact his thesis supervisor felt that the work was not suitable for the awarding of a thesis and Seldinger had to write another thesis, this time using his techniques in the field of percutaneous cholangiography. Seldinger became chief of radiology at the Mora Hospital in Sweden in 1967.

Early descriptions of angiography led to sophisticated techniques such as selective angiography being described with important contributions made by Alexander Margulis who went on to describe mesenteric angiography in the early 1960s. These pioneering studies were used to demonstrate sites of bleeding and people also realized that angiography could be used for intravenous thrombolysis.[7,8]

Charles Dotter and angioplasty

The concept of being able to dilate vessels using catheters and tubes made good advances following the experimentations of Charles T. Dotter (1920–1985).[9,10] In 1964 he described the technique of transluminal angioplasty. Dotter wrote a seminal paper in 1964 on this technique along with another great pioneering doctor, Melvin Judkins. Dotter was a true polymath who not only made major advances in radiology but also wrote one of the earliest papers on cardiac resuscitation in 1962 and was thought to be considerably ahead of his time. He was a pilot, a flier, and a mountain climber and had a wide range of interests including classical music, painting, photography, and outdoor living and was nominated for the Nobel Prize in Physiology or Medicine in 1978. Dotter is considered today as the father of interventional radiology. Figure 10.2 illustrates an inflated balloon during angioplasty of a popliteal artery in 1985. Cardiac angioplasty was pioneered by the work of the Swiss doctor Dr Andres Gruentzig who presented his animal studies of coronary angioplasty initially in 1976 and performed the first transluminous coronary angioplasty on an awake patient in Zurich in 1977.[11] This opened up the way for treating cardiac coronary problems with interventional imaging in radiology rather than open heart surgery. This pioneering breakthrough resulted in further improvements in treating coronary artery disease percutaneously and the subsequent decades saw the development of stents to keep these narrowed dilated vessels open.[12] Charles Dotter in fact developed the first stents, initially made with Nitinol. Subsequently throughout the 1980s a number of distinguished contributors including Palmaz and Strecker and others made major contributions in design structure and were involved in making these procedures a commonplace occurrence in hospital departments.[13,14]

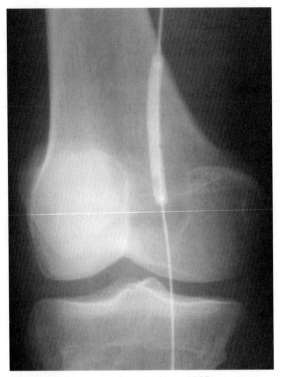

Fig. 10.2 Balloon inflation for popliteal angioplasty, 1985.
Image courtesy of Dr Adrian M.K. Thomas.

Non-angiographic intervention

Although angiography and technical developments associated with it were a primary driving force in the development of interventional imaging techniques, there were other developments in the field of interventional radiology. In the biliary system percutaneous transhepatic cholangiography (PTC) was first described in 1937. Figure 10.3 is a PTC from 1986 showing a stone at the lower end of a dilated bile duct. Extraction of retained common bile duct stones was in fact reported in 1962 by Burhenne. Over the next 20 years or so this technique was to become almost commonplace in radiological departments. Burhenne made great pioneering strides in this technique and built up a formidable experience with a success rate of around 95%.[15] In 1978 stents were introduced into the biliary system.[16] Stent technology continued

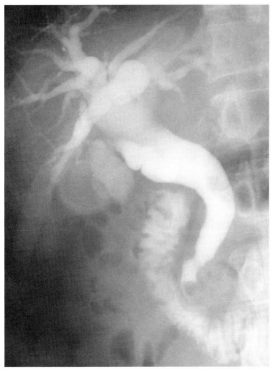

Fig. 10.3 A percutaneous transhepatic cholangiogram performed in 1986 showing a stone at the lower end of a dilated bile duct.

Image courtesy of Dr Adrian M.K. Thomas.

to develop throughout the 1980s and stents which can keep vessels and tubes open were not only used in the vascular system to keep arteries and veins patent but were also used to dilate narrowed airways in the tracheobronchial tree as well as in the urethra and in the colon and in the urinary tract to keep ureters patent.

In the renal tract nephrostomies were described by Goodwin, a nephrologist, as long ago as 1955.[17] This technique of introducing a needle into the dilated renal collecting system was used to treat hydronephrosis. The description of nephrostomy was reported in 1865 by Thomas Hillier from London who used this technique on a 4-year-old boy to drain abscesses although his early descriptions were not really looked at for over 100 years.

Image-guided biopsies and drainage

Interventional radiological techniques to drain abscesses became more commonplace in the 1970s and 1980s.[18,19] Initially ultrasound was used to guide catheter drainage of fluid collections within the body. In the 1980s computed tomography (CT) became the modality of choice in some situations and revolutionized the treatment of intra-abdominal fluid collections bypassing the need for surgery in these patients.

As radiological techniques became more and more sophisticated and more accurate at delineating lesions, more image-guided biopsies were performed.[20] These include image-guided biopsies of lung tumours, image-guided biopsies of liver lesions, and other abdominal lesions such as nodes and tumours could all be imaged first with a CT scan and then the CT scan could be used to guide biopsy needles such that more accurate precise localization of lesions could be effected and tissue samples obtained to enable an accurate diagnosis. Figure 10.4 shows a fine needle aspiration (FNA) of a defect in a lymph node opacified at lymphography in a patient with prostate cancer and performed in 1982. Figure 10.5 depicts an FNA of a lung nodule performed under fluoroscopic control in 1993. Lung biopsy under fluoroscopy has been replaced by CT-guided lung biopsy where a core of tissue can be obtained, permitting a more complex histological analysis by pathologists.

Modern interventional radiology

Today interventional techniques are used in all the organ systems in addition to routine angiographic demonstration of the arteries and angiographic interventions and stent placements. Embolization developed in the 1970s and Figure 10.6 illustrates a conventional hepatic arteriogram performed for liver embolization in 1984. The procedure was quite laborious since following an angiographic 'run' the radiologist had to wait several minutes for the film series taken in a serial changer to be processed. The flowering of modern interventional radiology has been possible due to a number of factors coming together. These were the development of image intensification followed by digital fluoroscopy and digital subtraction angiography, modern non-ionic contrast

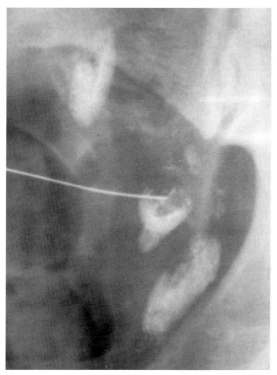

Fig. 10.4 A FNA of a defect in a lymph node opacified at lymphography, 1982.
Image courtesy of Dr Adrian M.K. Thomas.

media which were painless following injection, modern pre-shaped catheters and guidewires, and stents and endovascular coils. In the early days of catheter angiography the radiologist had to shape the catheter for selective angiography by hand. Radiologists are now able to apply these techniques within the carotid vascular system and also embolize arterial venous malformations in the brain. Embolization techniques are also used to stop bleeding from arteries and play an increasing role in the management of trauma in the abdominal system.[21] Interventional techniques are regularly used for biopsies and drainage procedures. In addition the biliary system can be approached both endoscopically (endoscopic retrograde cholangiopancreatogram) and transhepatically allowing appropriate stent placements for drainage of dilated biliary systems. Figure 10.7 illustrates a stent made by

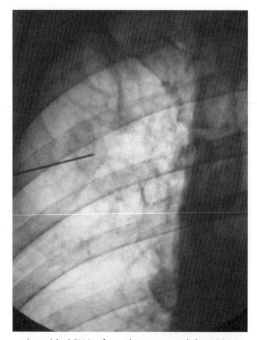

Fig. 10.5 Fluoroscopic-guided FNA of a pulmonary nodule, 1992.
Image courtesy of Dr Adrian M.K. Thomas.

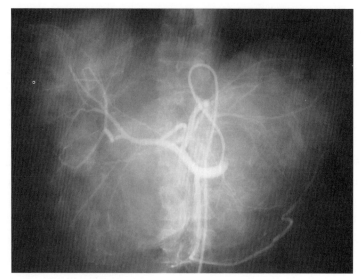

Fig. 10.6 Hepatic arteriogram for liver embolization in 1984.
Image courtesy of Dr Adrian M.K. Thomas.

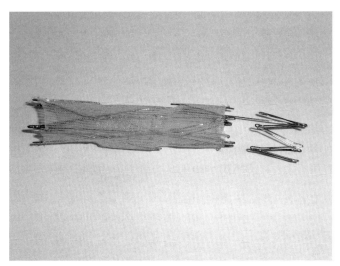

Fig. 10.7 A tracheal stent personally made by Gianturco.
Image courtesy of Dr Adrian M.K. Thomas.

Gianturco to treat a tracheal stenosis and covered by nylon stocking, also made by Gianturco. In the renal tract, interventional procedures allow the extraction of renal calculi and dilation of narrowed ureters. In the chest, interventions commonly performed include biopsies of the lung and stenting of the airways. Embolization of the bronchial arteries and arteriovenous malformations in the lungs can be employed as an alternative to thoracotomy and subsequent lobectomy. Future collaborations with surgical colleagues will result in more procedures, for example, aortic stent insertion being performed with minimally invasive interventional techniques, and radiologists will continue to play a leading part in these developments in the future.[22]

References

1. **Thomas, A.M.K., Banerjee, A.K., and Busch, U.** (2005). *Classic Papers in Modern Diagnostic Radiology*. Berlin: Springer Verlag.
2. **Burckhardt, H. and Müller, W.** (1921). Rontgendarstellung. *Deutshe Zeitschrift fur Chirurgie*, *162*, 168–197.
3. **Bruwer, A.J.** (1964). *Classic Descriptions in Diagnostic Radiology*. Springfield, IL: C.C. Thomas.
4. **Moniz, E.** (1927). L'encephalographie arterielle, son importance dans la localisation des tumours cerebrale. *Revue Neurologique*, *2*, 72–89.

5. **Sones, F.M., Jr., Sitirey, E.K., Proudeit, W.L., and Westcott, R.N.** (1959). Cine coronary angiography. *Circulation, 20*, 773–774.

6. **Seldinger, S.I.** (1953). Catheter replacement of the needle in percutaneous arteriography: a new technique. *Acta Radiologica, 39*, 368–376.

7. **Nusbaum, M. and Baum, S.** (1963). Radiographic demonstration of unknown sites of gastrointestinal bleeding. *Surgical Forum, 14*, 374–375.

8. **Johnson, A.J. and McCarty, W.R.** (1959). The lysis of artificially induced intravascular clots in man by intravenous infusions of streptokinase. *Journal of Clinical Investigation, 38*, 1627–1643.

9. **Dotter, C.T.** (1969). Transluminally-placed coilspring endarterial tube grafts: long-term patency in canine popliteal artery. *Investigative Radiology, 4*, 329–332.

10. **Dotter, C.T., Buschmann, R.W., McKinney, M.R., and Rosch, J.** (1983). Transluminal expandable nitinol coil stent grafting: preliminary report. *Radiology, 147*, 259–260.

11. **Gruntzig, A.** (1978). Transluminal dilatation of coronary artery stenosis. *Lancet, 1*, 263.

12. **Sigwart, U., Puel, J., Mirkovitch, V., et al.** (1987). Intravascular stents to prevent occlusion and restonosis after transluminal angioplasty. *New England Journal of Medicine, 316*, 701–706.

13. **Palmaz, J.C., Sibbitt, P.R., Reuter, S.R., et al.** (1985). Expandable intraluminal graft: preliminary study. *Radiology, 156*, 73–77.

14. **Gunther, R.W., Vorwerk, D., Bohndorf, K., et al.** (1989). Iliac and femoral artery stenosis and occlusion treatment with intravascular stents. *Radiology, 172*, 725–730.

15. **Burhenne, J.H.** (1974). Nonoperative roentgenologic instrumentation techniques of the postoperative biliary tract: treatment of biliary stricture and retained stones. *American Journal of Surgery, 128*, 111–117.

16. **Irving, J.D., Adam, A., Dick, R., Dondelinger, R.F., et al.** (1989). Expandable metallic stents: results of a European clinical trial. *Radiology, 172*, 321–326.

17. **Goodwin, W.E., Casey, W.C., and Wolf, W.** (1955). Percutaneous trocar (needle) nephrostomy in hydronephrosis. *Journal of the American Medical Association, 157* 891–894.

18. **Smith, E.H. and Bartrum, R.J.** (1974). Ultrasonically guided percutaneous aspiration of abscesses. *American Journal of Roentgenology, 122*, 308–312.

19. **Halasz, N.A. and Van Sonnenberg, E.** (1987). Drainage of intra-abdominal abscesses. Tactics and choices. *American Journal of Surgery, 146*(1), 112–115.

20. **Haaga, J.R. and Alfidi, R.J.** (1976). Precise biopsy localisation by CT. *Radiology, 118*, 603–607.

21. **Gianturco, C., Anderson, J.H., and Wallace, S.** (1975). Mechanical devices for arterial occlusion. *American Journal of Roentgenology, 124*, 428–435.

22. **Parodi, J.C., Palmaz, J.C., and Barone, H.D.** (1991). Transfemoral intraluminal graft implantation for abdominal aortic aneurysms. *Annals of Vascular Surgery, 5*, 491–499.

Chapter 11

A history of mammography

Following Röntgen's discovery of X-rays in 1895, the early clinical applications of this technique were predominantly confined to the skeletal system with particular emphasis on the bones. Initially it was not thought that X-rays would have a practical application in imaging soft tissues as clinicians felt that they could examine these areas clinically and obtain information by inspection and palpation.

The first person credited with imaging the breast using X-rays was an assistant professor of surgery in Berlin named Albert Solomon,[1] who in 1913 undertook the first examination of a breast cancer specimen using X-rays. The paper was published in the German journal *Archives of Clinical Surgery* and was entitled 'Contributions to the Pathology in Clinical Medicine of Breast Cancer'. Although this was the first demonstration of breast cancer in an excision specimen, it was not for several further years that examination of the breast in a living person would be carried out.

In 1926 an American from Rochester, New York, named Stafford Warren[2] published a report stating that he could see a reasonable outline of the breast while he was performing thoracic aortic fluoroscopy. In his series of 119 female patients he found 48 had breast cancer. In 1927 the German Otto Kleinschmidt[3] reported on his extensive experience of radiological examination of the breast in patients in Leipzig over many years. Patients with an uncertain diagnosis had undergone radiography and in addition surgical specimens obtained from the breast also underwent radiography. This was one of the earliest papers describing the role of radiography in the early detection of breast cancer. Other pioneers from Germany included Walter Mogul who in 1932 wrote a paper on the radiology of breast tumours.

Raoul Leborgne

Numerous papers were published in the 1930s, from as far afield as South America, by authors including Domingus (1930) and Baraldi (1935). At the same time workers from Paris including Espaillat (1933) were publishing their experience. It was Raoul Leborgne in 1935, working in Montevideo, Uruguay who made a major contribution to the field of breast imaging by differentiating between microcalcifications in benign disease from malignant disease. In 1943 he published an important monograph entitled 'The Radiology of the Lactiferous Duct System in the Normal and Pathological Mammary Gland'.[4] Leborgne stressed the importance of excellent radiographic techniques and in addition suggested a craniocaudal view for the mammogram in addition to the oblique view which had been the only view conducted until then. Leborgne emphasized his low-kilovoltage short-focus film distance and selected view techniques without screen films and breast compression in order to obtain the best possible images for diagnosing microcalcification.

In 1937 another pioneer, Gershon-Cohen from the USA,[5] published an important paper with radiological/pathological correlation. Gershon-Cohen's pathologist, Helen Ingleby, correlated for the first time both the anatomy and the pathology using the techniques of breast radiography. This team worked together for several years and in 1954 produced a study that showed that the accuracy of clinical examination was poor with clinical examination and palpation obtaining an inaccuracy of around 48% whereas radiological examination increased the accuracy to around 90%.[6]

Robert Egan and Charles Gros

In the 1950s, Robert Egan, working at the Tumour Institute of the University of Texas MD Anderson Hospital in Houston, made major technical contributions to what would constitute an optimal mammographic examination. He pioneered the high mA low kV technique and was the first to actually coin the term mammography for X-ray examination of the breast. He was a great early advocate of breast screening for the early detection of breast cancer. The French physicist Charles M. Gross also made technical advances in mammography by introducing the molybdenum anode tube which was the first tube dedicated to mammography.

Siemens in the 1960s also made contributions to the field of mammography by improving the low-radiation technique with a special X-ray tube with a rotating anode and a thinner glass window.

Numerous technical developments were produced in the 1970s and 1980s. More refinements of microcalcification analysis were introduced in the 1970s by Marton Lanyi from Germany and colleagues. Mammography was not an exact science and difficulty in analysing and interpreting mammograms were soon realized in the 1960s with major contributions in this field made by John Wolfe who was to write an article in 1966 entitled 'Mammography Errors in Diagnosis'. Wolfe, from the USA, was also an advocate of the new technique introduced in the 1960s of xeroradiography.

Breast screening

In the 1970s, advocates of mass screening for the early detection of cancers came to the forefront. In Sweden in 1978 mass screening was introduced and Laszlo Tabar[7] from the Faloun Central Hospital compared the deaths from breast cancer in two Swedish counties 20 years before and after screening. This was an important study that showed that women who had screening had a reduced risk of dying from breast cancer. Since then several countries have adopted breast screening as a health screening tool. In the UK breast screening was started in the late 1980s after the Forrest report. Controversies remain regarding the benefits and disadvantages of screening.

Digital mammography

Undoubtedly technical developments have driven forward the use of mammography in the early detection of breast cancer and this has saved many lives over the years. More recently digital mammography was introduced by Smathers and co-workers in 1986. This has now replaced

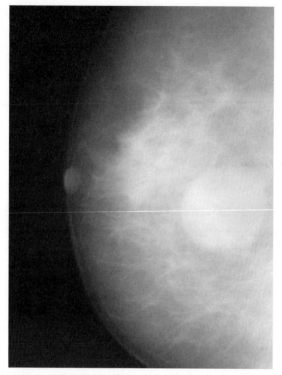

Fig. 11.1 Breast cysts on shown on conventional film mammography in 1976.
Image courtesy of Dr Adrian M.K. Thomas.

the screen film image in most centres. Digital mammography is more sensitive at detecting microcalcification in the breast tissue and enables earlier detection of smaller, early cancers. Figure 11.1 illustrates breast cysts shown on conventional mammography in 1976.

Breast biopsy and one-stop clinics

In the 1970s non-palpable breast lesions were localized with stereotactic guidance with pioneering work by Nordstrom[8] from Sweden in 1977. Parker[9] pioneered the role of ultrasound to guide biopsy in the 1990s in the USA. Today ultrasound-guided and stereotactic-guided biopsies are routine practice. It is the refinements in ultrasound machines that have occurred over the last 20 years that have made more accurate localization of breast lesions in younger patients possible, thus raising the diagnostic accuracy of imaging over clinical examination. Today in breast clinics triple assessment is carried out which involves clinical examination, imaging, and biopsy of suspicious areas, to detect early malignancy.[10] Newer techniques of magnetic resonance imaging (MRI) have also been used as an adjunct to help increase the accuracy of breast cancer detection and are the latest in the armamentarium of diagnostic modalities available for the detection of breast cancer.

Pelvimetry

Interest in the assessment of the female pelvis in pregnant women is not a new phenomenon. Pelvimetry using an instrument, the pelvimeter, was invented in the late 1700s by the Frenchman Jean Louis Baudeloque (1746–1810). The pelvimeter was shaped like pelvis forceps and the opening of the handles allowed measurements to be read off, thus enabling the obstetrician to assess which patients were more likely to obstruct during labour due to abnormalities in the pelvic shape and size. An example of the pelvimeter may be seen in the Science Museum in London.

With the discovery of X-rays, imaging in the assessment of the female pelvis became a possibility and for many years relied on plain radiographic assessment of the pelvic inlet and outlet. Based on these assessments four types of pelvis were characterized, including gynaecoid, which was the ideal shape for the best chances of a normal vaginal delivery, and android, anthropoid, and platypelloid pelvises. Radiographic assessment of the pelvis alongside clinical assessment helped the obstetrician to plan obstetric care and the form of delivery that would safely be possible in each patient. Figure 11.2 is an example of conventional pelvimetry performed for a breech presentation in 1985.

X-ray pelvimetry was often used to assess obstetric patients for normal labour in the 1950s and 1960s but by the early 1970s studies were being published to show that this was not necessarily a useful procedure. Computed tomography (CT) was a new tool in the 1970s that could also be used to assess the pelvic inlet and outlet. Radiation dosages with these techniques were high and only complicated cases were investigated in this way. Clearly, however, because of the radiation involved,

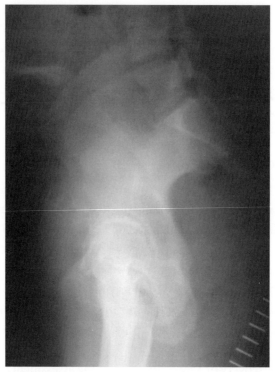

Fig. 11.2 Erect lateral pelvimetry in 1985 for breech presentation of the baby.
Image courtesy of Dr Adrian M.K. Thomas.

these techniques soon fell into disuse. In the 1980s with the advances in sonography, and a decade later with the advent of MRI, the technique of plain X-ray pelvimetry and CT pelvimetry was almost rendered obsolete in the assessment of the pelvic inlet and outlet in the management of obstetric patients undergoing potential labour.

Gynaecography

Before cross-sectional imaging techniques including CT, MRI, and ultrasound were available, imaging of the female reproductive organs was difficult. One method of performing visualization of the internal female reproductive organs included the technique of gynaecography (Figure 11.3) where air was introduced into the peritoneum creating a pneumoperitoneum. This enabled radiographic visualization of the

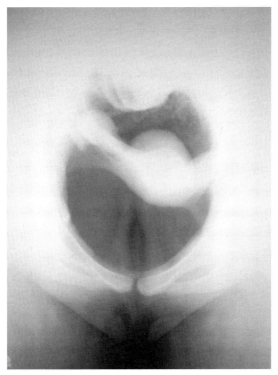

Fig. 11.3 Pelvic gynaecography outlining the pelvic organs.
Image courtesy of Dr Adrian M.K. Thomas.

reproductive structures. This technique was popular in the 1960s. Gynaecography enabled ovarian visualization and enabled a diagnosis of ovarian failure and gonadal dysgenesis. The technique has now become practically obsolete due to better imaging techniques with ultrasound, CT, and MRI which are all now in the diagnostic armamentarium of radiologists and gynaecologists along with direct laparoscopic visualization itself which has become routine practice in the last 20 years or so.

Development of ultrasound and MRI in relation to imaging in women

Since Donald's pioneering study on ultrasound, scanning machines have improved considerably in resolution and accuracy enabling much improved care of the obstetric patient with regard to the evaluation of the fetus from conception to delivery. In addition, advances in transvaginal scanning in the 1980s onwards had led to a far more accurate assessment of the ovaries and in particularly to assessment of the infertile patient. These techniques have greatly influenced the practice of obstetrics and gynaecology and have led to a marked improvement in the quality of care delivered to those women all around the world who have access to these technologies.

Ultrasound scanning has resulted in the better detection of antenatal abnormalities and has helped guide the obstetrician as to the best mode of delivery, enabling higher standards of care to be provided for female patients and their newborns. More recently, MRI has also been used in more complicated cases to assess the obstetric patient, and in particular to assess placental abnormalities.

In the last 10 years or so the improvements in MRI scanners and a greater access to these technologies has resulted in better and more accurate staging of gynaecological malignancies (using both MRI and CT scanning) and this has played a major part in the improvement and outcome of patients.

Unfortunately one of the by-products of ultrasound scanning has been the inappropriate use of antenatal assessment of the fetus for the selective abortion of the female fetus in certain cultures and countries around the world. Nowhere has the ethics of medical practice and high technology and obstetric care and cultural sensitivity been intertwined in greater complexity.

The social impact of ultrasound

Since Donald's discovery of ultrasound and the subsequent improvements in instrument design and reduction in instrument size and complexity, ultrasound has played a huge role in the diagnostic armamentarium of health workers throughout the world. Even in poorer countries it is possible to have ultrasound machines to facilitate a more accurate diagnosis for a wide variety of conditions; abdominal, obstetric, and gynaecological problems have been helped greatly by this new technology. The social impact of this cannot be underestimated. Improvements in health outcomes are now possible with relatively modest investment in technology. Health workers can be trained around the world to utilize these machines for the benefit of patients in their communities. The management of acute abdominal conditions has been improved. Obstetric care has been markedly improved, making pregnancy safer. Figure 11.4 illustrates obstetric ultrasound from 1985. As mentioned, one of the sad side effects is the selective abortion of female fetuses in certain cultures but several governments are trying to control the inappropriate use of ultrasound for these purposes.

With greater refinement in techniques, ultrasound machines have become more portable and can be used at the bedside, thus facilitating an even more accurate diagnosis among really ill patients on hospital wards and intensive care units. This trend is surely likely to increase in the future and we shall see a wider variety and range of medical and healthcare personnel using ultrasound for investigative purposes which no doubt will raise questions about whether all the personnel are being appropriately trained to handle these machines and make appropriate diagnoses. Issues of training and turf wars are likely to be paramount over the coming years what with an increasing ageing population and

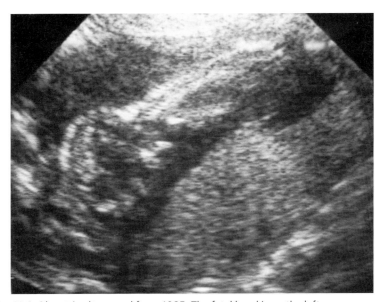

Fig. 11.4 Obstetric ultrasound from 1985. The fetal head is on the left.
Image courtesy of Dr Adrian M.K. Thomas.

increasing usage of high-technology imaging facilities, not only in the Western world but in developing nations too.

References

1. **Salomon, A.** (1913). Beitrage zur pathologie und klinik der mammakarzinome. *Archivfiir Klinische Chirurgie, 103,* 573–668.

2. **Warren, S.L.** (1930). A roentgenologic study of the breast. *American Journal of Roentgenology and Radiation Therapy, 24,* 113–124.

3. **Kleinschmidt, O.** (1927). Brustdruse. In Zweife, P.E., Payr, E., and Hirzel, S. (Eds), *Die Klinik der bösartigen Geschwülste,* pp. 5–90. Leipzig: Hirzel.

4. **Leborgne, R.** (1943). *Estudio Radiológico del Sistema Canalicular de la Glándula Mamaria Normal y Patológica.* Montivideo: Primera Edicao.

5. **Gershon-Cohen, J. and Colcher, A.E.** (1937). Evaluation of roentgen diagnosis of early carcinoma of breast. *Journal of the American Medical Association, 108,* 867–871.

6. **Gershon-Cohen, J., Ingleby, H., Hermel, M.B.,** *et al.* (1954). Accuracy of pre-operative x-ray diagnosis of breast tumour. *Surgery, 35,* 766–771.

7. **Tabár, L., Fagerburg, C.J.G., Gad, A.,** *et al.* (1985). Reduction in mortality from breast cancer after mass screening with mammography. Randomised trial from the Breast Cancer Screening Working Group of the Swedish National Board of Health and Welfare. *Lancet, 1,* 829–832.

8. **Norderstrom, B.** (1977). Stereotactic screw needle biopsy of non-palpable breast lesions. In Logan W. and Muntz, E.P. (Eds), *Breast Carcinoma: The Radiologist's Expanded Role,* pp. 313–318. New York, NY: Wiley.

9. **Parker, S.H., Lovin, J.D., Jobe, W.E.,** *et al.* (1990). Stereotactic breast biopsy with a biopsy gun. *Radiology, 176,* 741–747.

10. **Wolfe, J.N.** (1966). Mammography: errors in diagnosis. *Radiology, 87,* 214–219.

Chapter 12

Nuclear medicine and radioactivity: from nuclear biology to molecular imaging

Nuclear imaging started in the late 1940s when nuclear reactors started to produce radioactive isotopes that could be used as tracers for diagnosis and agents for therapy and its history has been recently reviewed by Henry Wagner.[1] Henri Becquerel had discovered his Becquerel rays in 1896 which was the year after Wilhelm Röntgen had discovered his rays but the medical applications of the two phenomena were very different. X-rays could be put to use immediately because the apparatus was available in many physics laboratories and the technique needed was relatively simple. However, radioactivity was an entirely different matter and radioactive elements were difficult to both locate and isolate. It was only following the development of the cyclotron and nuclear reactors that radioisotopes could be produced that could have a medical use other than for therapy. The cyclotron was invented in 1931 by Ernest Lawrence in California and the first cyclotron for biomedical research was opened in 1940 in Cambridge, Massachusetts. The original nuclear reactor was first made to work successfully in a squash rackets court under a sports stadium in Chicago on 2 December 1942.

Although the existence of atoms had been proposed by Democritus over 2000 years ago, it was Robert Boyle (1627–1691) who was the first atomic scientist to realize that there were many different types of atom (or first principles) of which matter is composed. John Dalton (1766–1844) took the first modern steps forward and proposed that:

Atoms are separate real material particles that cannot be subdivided.
Atoms of the same element are similar in all respect and equal in weight.
Atoms of different elements have different properties.
'Compounds' are formed by the union of atoms of different elements in simple numerical proportions.[2]

Henri Becquerel and the Curies

Henri Becquerel (1852–1908)

Antoine Henri Becquerel illustrated in a painting by Katie Golding (Figure 12.1) was born in Paris on 15 December 1852 and died at Le Croisic on 25 August 1908. He was a member of a distinguished French scientific family. Becquerel was appointed to the Chair of Applied Physics at the Conservatoire des Arts et Métiers in Paris, taking over from his father Alexander Edmond Becquerel.

In 1892 he was appointed as Professor of Applied Physics at the Paris Museum and became a Professor at the Polytechnic in 1895. Becquerel was interested in phosphorescence throughout his career and in 1896 he discovered the phenomenon of natural radioactivity.

In January 1896 H. Poincaré informed Becquerel of the discovery of X-rays by Wilhelm Röntgen. In February he noted the effect of uranyl

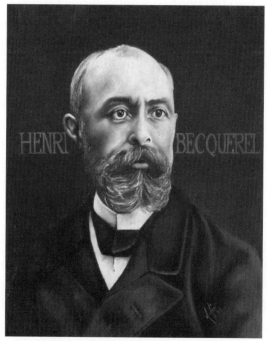

Fig. 12.1 Henri Becquerel by the artist Katie Golding.
Image courtesy of Dr Adrian M.K. Thomas.

and phosphate salts on photographic glass and in March he demonstrated the discharge of electrified bodies by the new phenomenon. When a new discovery is made it is interesting to observe that others are also independently investigating the same area, for example, Wilhelm Röntgen and William Crookes in X-rays and Charles Darwin and Alfred Wallace in evolutionary theory. The British physicist Silvanus Thompson had noted the action of uranium on photographic glass on 27 February 1896 which was a mere 3 days after the publication by Henri Becquerel of his discovery in *Comptes Rendus* of the 24 February of that year (Figure 12.2).

For his discovery Becquerel was awarded half of the Nobel Prize for Physics in 1903 'in recognition of the extraordinary services he has rendered by his discovery of spontaneous radioactivity,' sharing it with the Curies. It was actually Marie Curie who coined the word radioactivity. In spite of the many contributions of Antoine Henri Becquerel, he remains less well known when compared with Wilhelm Conrad Röntgen and with Marie and Pierre Curie. As yet no full length biography has been written of Becquerel in English. In *Cultures of Creativity: The Centennial Exhibition of the Nobel Prize*, for 1903 there is only mention of the Curies and no mention that Becquerel had received half of the Nobel Prize and that the Curies had received a quarter each. Becquerel was only 55 when he died of a sudden heart attack at the summer resort of Le Croisic, when he had recently been elected as Président de l'Académie des Science and then Secrétaire perpetual pour les Sciences Physiques. Henri Becquerel married Lucie Jamin in 1877 (the daughter of a well-known physicist) and sadly she had died in 1878, 1 month after the birth of their son Jean who also became a physicist.

It is not surprising therefore that the first non-SI unit for radiation was named after the Curies and not after Becquerel. This was corrected in 1975 when the General Conference on Weights and Measures (CGPM) decided to honour Henri Becquerel by adopting the special name of Becquerel, Bq, for the SI derived unit of activity. This proposal had been made by the International Commission for Radiation Units and Measurements (ICRU) and accepted by the Consultative Committee for Units (CCU) in 1974.

(501)

qui émettent des radiations fluorescentes de couleur jaune verdâtre peuvent impressionner la plaque photographique à travers les corps opaques.

» Les résultats contradictoires ci-dessus s'expliquent donc très bien en tenant compte des faits signalés par MM. Charles Henry, Niewenglowski, et surtout par notre confrère M. Henri Becquerel dans les dernières séances. Les corps fluorescents émettent des radiations jouissant des propriétés des rayons X conformément à l'hypothèse de notre confrère M. Poincaré.

» De tous ces faits il résulte que le rôle des rayons cathodiques dans les expériences de Röntgen semble se borner à exciter la fluorescence du verre spécial composant l'ampoule de Crookes. »

PHYSIQUE. — *Sur les radiations invisibles émises par les corps phosphorescents.* Note de M. HENRI BECQUEREL.

« Dans la dernière séance, j'ai indiqué sommairement les expériences que j'avais été conduit à faire pour mettre en évidence les radiations invisibles émises par certains corps phosphorescents, radiations qui traversent divers corps opaques pour la lumière.

» J'ai pu étendre ces observations, et, bien que je me propose de continuer et de développer l'étude de ces phénomènes, leur actualité me conduit à exposer, dès aujourd'hui, les premiers résultats que j'ai obtenus.

» Les expériences que je rapporterai ont été faites avec les radiations émises par des lamelles cristallines de sulfate double d'uranyle et de potassium

$$[SO^4(UO)K + H^2O],$$

corps dont la phosphorescence est très vive et la durée de persistance lumineuse inférieure à $\frac{1}{100}$ de seconde. Les caractères des radiations lumineuses émises par cette substance ont été étudiés autrefois par mon père et j'ai eu, depuis, l'occasion de signaler quelques particularités intéressantes que présentent ces radiations lumineuses.

» On peut vérifier très simplement que les radiations émises par cette substance, quand elle est exposée au soleil ou à la lumière diffuse du jour, traversent, non seulement des feuilles de papier noir, mais encore divers métaux, par exemple une plaque d'aluminium et une mince feuille de cuivre. J'ai fait notamment l'expérience suivante :

» Une plaque Lumière, au gélatino-bromure d'argent, a été enfermée dans un châssis opaque en toile noire, fermé d'un côté par une plaque

Fig. 12.2 The first description of what became known as radioactivity by Henri Becquerel in *Comptes Rendus* 24 February 1896.

Reprinted from *Comptes Rendus de l'Académie des Sciences, 122*, p. 501, session of 24 February 1896.

Marie (1867–1934) and Pierre (1859–1906) Curie

Marie Curie was a remarkable woman and her life story is one of the inspirational stories of humanity.[2] The biography of Marie written by her daughter Eve is one of the greatest biographies of the 20th century and new biographies continue to appear.[3] Her partnership with Pierre Curie was one of the greatest scientific collaborations of all time. Marie Curie was a full professor at a time when it was very unusual for universities to employ women at all. She was also a partner with her daughter Irène who became a physicist. It was Marie Curie's daughter Irène and her husband Frederick Joliot who discovered artificial radioactivity in 1934 when they creating radioactive nitrogen from boron, radioactive isotopes of phosphorus from aluminium, and silicon from magnesium. For this achievement, in 1935 the Joliot-Curies were awarded the Nobel Prize for Chemistry. After the Second World War, Frederick Joliot started France's nuclear power program and worked for international peace.

It is debatable whether the discovery that earned the 1903 Nobel Prize for Physics was in the fields of chemistry or of physics. The winner of the Nobel Prize for Chemistry for 1903 was reported as saying that the discovery of radium was the single most important discovery in that subject for the previous century. The award citation does not make specific mention of the discovery of either radium or polonium and so the possibility of a further Nobel Prize for Chemistry remained. This proved to be the case and on 11 November 1911 Marie Curie received a telegram telling her that she was to be awarded the Nobel Prize for Chemistry which was to be in recognition of her services in the advancement of chemistry by the discovery of the elements radium and polonium, by the isolation of radium, and the study of the nature and compounds of this remarkable element. There has been much discussion over the years about this second Nobel Prize since the work being rewarded was essentially the same as that which had been recognized in the 1903 award. It is possible that part of the motivation for the award was to show support for her at a time of intense personal attack, related partly to the scandal of her relationship with fellow physicist Paul Langevin which had cost her a place in the French Academy of Sciences. At the Nobel Award Ceremony on 10 December 1911 it was explained that the reason for giving her the second Nobel Prize for the same work was because of the major significance of radium and that the study of radium was important in two areas. First, radium showed that the long-standing view that atoms were unchanging was false and that one element could transform itself into another. This was the new alchemy and Marie Curie paid tribute to Ernest Rutherford in her acceptance speech. Second, there were the major medical uses of radium in the treatment of cancer.

Pierre Curie had been killed in a tragic street accident in Paris on 19 April 1906 and Marie was appointed to his chair. In her first lecture to the physics course at the Sorbonne in Paris on 5 November 1906, the recently widowed Marie Sklodowsa Curie spoke the following words 'When one considers the progress that has been made in physics in the past ten years, one is surprised at the advance that has taken place in our ideas concerning electricity and matter'.[4] Her words are true and if we believe that we now live in a time of great scientific change then there were even more profound changes in the decade leading up to this November 1906 lecture. When Röntgen discovered X-rays in 1895 the whole edifice of classical physics had seemed so stable and sure. The discovery of X-rays had been followed rapidly in 1896 by the discovery of radioactivity and by 1906 there had been a profound change in our understanding of physics and modern physics had been born.

Radium

Radium was seen as a wonder element and produced a sense of hope, particularly in the treatment of cancer. Unfortunately it was believed that since radium was helpful in treating cancer it would also help in improving health in a more general way. There was a common idea in the early 20th century that radium and radiation were beneficial in low doses and indeed there is some experimental evidence for this. Radium could be used in creams, shampoo, and toothpaste, and for drinking. Radium for drinking to improve health and the illustration (Figure 12.3) shows an original 1935 radium emanator for producing radioactive water for drinking. The 'Radium-Émanateur' was distributed by

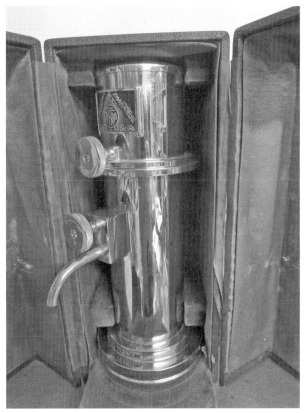

Fig. 12.3 The infamous 'Radium-Émanateur' from 1935 used for producing radioactive drinking water.
Image courtesy of Dr Adrian M.K. Thomas.

the Office Français du Radium and was recommended for many uses including gout, rheumatism, and circulatory and digestive problems. The accompanying certificate from the Institut du Radium (Laboratoire Curie) confirms the radioactivity in the apparatus. The emanation from the device could be taken as a drink or used in a bath. In Britain such emanators were manufactured by Radium Utilities Ltd and the Radium-Vita company. Until the mid-1950s the Radium-Vita manufactured creams and ointments containing radium.

Unfortunately the use of these emanators was not without considerable risk. The saddest case was that of the Pittsburgh millionaire Eben McButrney Byers who was recommended to drink Radiothor in 1928. He became a keen advocate of the rejuvenating treatment and gave it to his friends and also to his horses. He developed signs of radium poisoning and died at the age of 52 of a brain abscess and aplastic anaemia in 1932.

Such quack medical use of radium should not make us forget the real benefit of radium when used correctly. However, it does illustrate the uncritical and positive attitude to radiation in the pre-war years. A further radium disaster was the fate of the radium dial painters who ingested radium because of a habit of licking their brushes to make them into a point. The problem with the use of radium, both medically and commercially, is its long half-life. Radium-226 has a half-life of 1600 years which results in significant environmental issues for disposal. There was a Second World War airfield in Dalgety Bay in Fife, Scotland where many old aircraft were dismantled and incinerated. There is now contamination of the beach from the radium used in the dials of the old aircraft and erosion of the landfill site has resulted in contamination of the beach.

The influence of nuclear medicine in the Second World War

All of the positive attitudes to radiation were to change in 1945 with the tragedies of Hiroshima and Nagasaki. The public perception of radiation altered and radiation became irrevocably linked to the atomic bomb with all its negative associations. This fear was to increase in the 1950s and 1960s with the tensions of the Cold War. The Cold War encouraged the fear of nuclear weapons and the public mind did not separate this from peaceful uses of radiation. However, part of the problem for the public was that all aspects of radiation seemed to be veiled in State secrecy and this created a climate of suspicion. This was to continue with the accidents at Windscale in 1957, Three Mile Island in 1979, Chernobyl in 1986, and Fukushima in 2011, and others.

Many doctors were interested in the new artificial radioisotopes that could be produced by a cyclotron or nuclear reactor. By 1946 J.S. Mitchell from Cambridge was already considering the possible medical applications of radioisotopes to medicine as soon as they would become available. Mitchell saw the radioactive isotopes as being used as tracers to study metabolic processes, as radioactive sources for therapy, and as agents with therapeutic properties that were related to their selective concentration in body tissues.[3]

The concept of using radioactive material as a biological tracer had been described first by the Hungarian George Hevesy (1885–1966) who received the Nobel Prize in 1943. In 1923 Hevesy co-discovered hafnium. There was a perceived gap in Mendeleev's periodic table for an element with 72 protons and, using a sample from the mineralogical museum in Copenhagen, Hevesy found a characteristic X-ray spectral recording proving the presence of the new element. This earned him jointly with Dirk Coster the 1943 Nobel Prize in Chemistry.

Hevesy had worked with Ernest Rutherford on radium D (an isotope of lead). In experiments in 1913 Hevesy mixed a known amount of pure radium D with a known amount of a lead salt 'and to follow up the paths of the lead atoms using radium D . . . as an indicator'.[1] Using a naturally occurring radioisotope of lead Hersey studied the distribution of lead in the broad bean plant in a series of classic experiments. This is the tracer principle, allowing us to follow molecules in chemical reactions and as Henry Wagner wrote, 'It is as if a molecule emitted a radiosignal telling us what it was doing at all times'.[1] This is the basis of our modern nuclear medicine and of molecular imaging.

The first tracer studies in humans were carried out by Herman Blumgart and co-workers in Boston in 1925. Blumgart injected a solution of radium C into a patient's right arm and measured the time it took for the radioactivity to be detectable in the left arm using a Wilson cloud chamber. This measured the circulation time and this was measurable and independent of the amount of radioisotope injected.

Atoms for peace and Joseph Rotblat

In order to counteract the negative aspects of radiation following the bombing of Japan an 'Atoms for Peace' programme was started following the Second World War to educate the public about the beneficial aspects of radiation.

A key figure in the UK was Joseph Rotblat (1908–2005).[4] Rotblat was born in Poland and became a British citizen, going to Liverpool University in 1939 to work with James Chadwick who had discovered the neutron. In 1944 Rotblat then accompanied Chadwick's group to the USA to work on the Manhattan Project with the aim of building an atomic bomb. While in the USA Rotblat came to the belief that on moral grounds he had to stop working on the application of nuclear physics to the development of weapons of immense destructive power and turn his attention to medical applications. As a result he was the only scientist to quit the Manhattan Project and he was viewed with considerable suspicion. He realized that the general public was ignorant of the peaceful applications of atomic energy. In 1946 he was involved with others in the UK in setting up the Atomic Scientists Association. The members included scientists, many of whom had been involved during the war in the atomic energy projects in Britain, Canada, and the USA, and a major aim of the association was to bring before the public of the UK the true facts about atomic energy and the implications of its use. Rotblat and the Association were involved in a travelling exhibition called 'The Atom Train' and Rotblat was responsible for obtaining funding from the government. In early 1947 planning for The Atom Train was started and all the exhibition material was assembled in the Physics Department at University of Liverpool. The Train consisted of two large goods carriages and toured 26 railway stations, and the coaches would stay for between 3 and 6 days on a platform with members of the Association giving talks and physics students acting as guides and lecturers. The train was active for 168 days in 1947 to 1948 and exceeded by far the expectations of the Association. The topics covered included all aspects of radiation. Maps were displayed that would show the visitor the effects of a bomb dropped on central London, showing the range and areas of destruction, and there was a similar map of the local area of the town that the train visited. The use of radioisotopes in medicine for diagnostics and treatment were clearly outlined with illustrations, and the use of radioactive tracers in agriculture and industry were explained. At the end the visitors were presented with the choices that were open to them with the possibility of good or evil, either construction or destruction.

As an example of constructive use, in 1947 the physicist Joseph Rotblat and the physician George Ansell, both at Liverpool, demonstrated a retrosternal thyroid using radioactive iodine and external counting. They used the first sample of iodine-131 that had been produced on GLEEP (Graphite Low energy Experimental Pile) at the UK's first nuclear reactor located at Harwell. There were no chemical facilities at Harwell so the sample of irradiated tellurium was brought to Liverpool on Sunday 28 September 1947 and the chemical separation was made in the University Department of Biochemistry by George Ansell and his colleagues. The paper[5] has a clinical introduction and then described their initial studies using a naturally-occurring radioactive source. The end-window GM4 Geiger counter was illustrated and their complete apparatus described (Figure 12.4). They mounted the collimated counter on an X-ray stand. The intrathoracic thyroid tissue was outlined accurately in this first clinical scan in the UK (Figure 12.5). The authors indicated that radioiodine could also be used for the treatment of hyperthyroidism and selected cases of thyroid carcinoma. This paper was the first on many to appear in the field that would become known as 'nuclear medicine'. The clinical use of radioactive isotopes of iodine had been pioneered in the USA where, in 1936, John Lawrence had carried out experiments using iodine-131. Lawrence had obtained his from his brother E.O. Lawrence who had invented the cyclotron.

Joseph Rotblat was appointed professor of physics at St. Bartholomew's Hospital in London in 1950, retiring in 1978. After the Second World War his work on nuclear fallout made a major contribution to the partial nuclear test ban treaty. He was a signatory of the Russell–Einstein manifesto and was the General Secretary of the Pugwash Conferences on Science and World Affairs (<http://www.pugwash.org>) from its origin until 1973, becoming its President in 1988. In 1995, with the Pugwash Conferences, he received the Nobel Peace Prize for his efforts towards nuclear disarmament. His Presidential Address of 1972 to the British Institute of Radiology (BIR) is important for everyone interested in the ethical and moral implications of science. Rotblat believed that both individually and collectively as members of the institute (the BIR) they could contribute to the effort to save civilization and help in

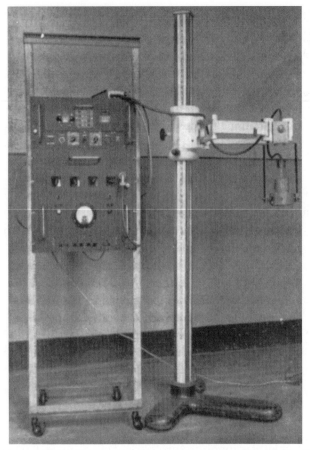

Fig. 12.4 Mounted GM4 Geiger counter as used by Ansell and Rotblat in 1948.

Reproduced with permission from G. Ansell and J. Rotblat, Radioactive iodine and a diagnostic aid for intrathoracic goitre, *British Journal of Radiology*, Vol. *21*, No. 251, pp. 552–558, Copyright © 1948 The British Institute of Radiology.

creating conditions in which man would live not only in better health but also in peace and security.

Early nuclear medicine

The new discipline of nuclear medicine was in its infancy in the 1950s but was growing rapidly.[6,7] In 1950 the *British Journal of Radiology* published Supplement No. 2, 'Some Applications of Nuclear Physics to Medicine', by W.V. Mayneord and this became a standard text for the next 10 years.

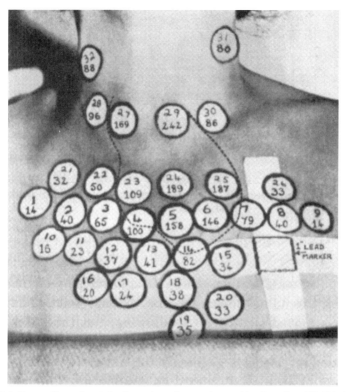

Fig. 12.5 The outline of an intrathoracic goitre performed by Ansell and Rotblat in 1948.

Reproduced with permission from G. Ansell and J. Rotblat, Radioactive iodine and a diagnostic aid for intrathoracic goitre, *British Journal of Radiology*, Vol. *21*, No. 251, pp. 552–558, Copyright © 1948 The British Institute of Radiology.

Mayneord had given a series of lectures to the BIR on this topic and the term 'nuclear medicine' is a contraction of Mayneord's title. A symposium was held in the UK in 1950 on the diagnostic and therapeutic use of radioactive isotopes and the papers appeared in the *British Journal of Radiology*. They are a fascinating account of knowledge at the start of a new discipline. Norman Veall from Hammersmith wrote on the measurement of radioactivity and there is an illustration of the measurement of thyroid uptake of radioiodine. Veall drew isocount contours of the radioisotope distributions in the thyroid gland. C.P. Haig from Bristol Mental Hospitals looked at clinical diagnosis and investigated thyroid function and performed early brain analysis. Joseph Rotblat and

R. Marcus from Liverpool had examined a case of multiple melanoma and considered whether internal irradiation from a radioactive isotope might be of value in treatment by being concentrated in the tumour. Alastair MacGregor from Sheffield assessed radioiodine in the diagnosis of thyrotoxicosis building on the work of Edward Pochin. Pochin had treated his first patient with thyroid cancer in June 1949 and had introduced 'profile counting' to localize secondary deposits and monitor the response to therapy. In August 1951 Edward Pochin gave a full report on radioiodine treatment in thyroid cancer and by this time over 300 patients had been treated with radioiodine. R.J. Walton described the use of radioactive isotopes at the Royal Cancer Hospital where they had been putting radioactive sodium into the bladder for bladder and using radioactive phosphorus for polycythaemia rubra vera. Finally R.G. Blomfield from Sheffield gave his experience of radioiodine in thyroid disease.

The rectilinear scanner

The early nuclear medicine studies were performed using a Geiger–Müller counter.[8] It was soon realized that if the counter was collimated it would only receive radiation from a small part of the field of interest. The probe could be moved by hand sequential over the field of interest and a map of count rates could be produced. This was hard work since the lead used for collimation was heavy and the pioneer Keith Halnan described how his own biceps developed considerably in the course of this type of work!

It is perhaps no accident that Atkinson Morley's Hospital in South London was chosen as a site for the EMI scanner in the late 1960s since there was a history of interest in innovative approaches to imaging at that hospital. In the early 1950s the neurosurgeon Wylie McKissock, who was later to work with James Ambrose, was collaborating with the Royal Marsden Hospital in developing 'isotope encephalography' since, unlike ventriculography and arteriography, there was no mortality and practically no discomfort to the patient. In a similar manner to computed tomography (CT), a special building was erected at Atkinson Morley's Hospital. There a skull survey was performed using an uncollimated detector and then collimated detectors in two planes at right angles in order to locate the abnormality in space. The results were not very encouraging but they were able to give advice on methods to reduce sources of error.

From the early 1950s automatic systems were introduced with movement of the detector in relation to the patient and this could linked to a printer to give a dot display, and the Geiger–Müller counter was replaced with a scintillation counter. This was accomplished by Benedict Cassen in 1951. There were many systems devised and in 1961 John Mallard, J.F. Fowler, and Maurice Sutton from Hammersmith Hospital used a scanner that moved the couch with stationary detectors and demonstrated brain tumours using radioactive arsenic. By the mid-1960s the technique had improved and brain scintigraphy with the rectilinear scanner was being performed more routinely. The nuclear medicine scans were of low resolution compared to the high-resolution radiographic images of the time but the results were obtainable without the invasive radiodiagnostic procedures that were performed so frequently. Figure 12.6 illustrates a radionuclide thyroid scan performed on a rectilinear scanner.

Hal Anger and his camera

Hal O. Anger (1920–2005) was a major figure in the development of nuclear medicine instrumentation. He obtained a BSc degree in 1943 from the University of California, Berkley, and then from 1943 to 1946 undertook research on radar at the Radio Research Laboratory of Harvard University. It is interesting to recollect that Godfrey Hounsfield was working on radar at the same time in the UK. Following the war Anger worked at the Donner Laboratory at the University of California, Berkeley. His first major new instrument was a scintillation well counter to measure iron-59 and replacing the Geiger–Müller beta counters that he had devised in 1950. Following the description of the rectilinear scanner Anger immediately set about devising an improved system. This was his 'Mark 1 Whole-Body Scanner' of 1953 and consisted of a linear arrangement of ten counters. The scanner moved over the patient to produce a whole-body scan and was particularly used to

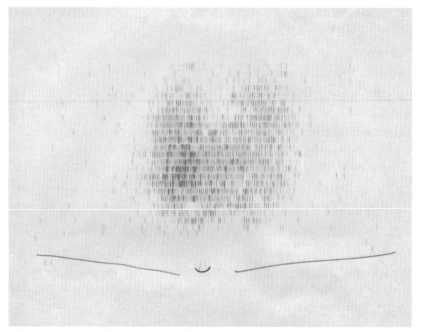

Fig. 12.6 Radionuclide thyroid scan performed on a rectilinear scanner.
Image courtesy of Dr Adrian M.K. Thomas.

detect functioning metastatic disease from thyroid carcinoma. Anger was, however, convinced that the best solution for imaging would be stationary devices in preference to a moving collimated detector. The advantage of a stationary detector is that it would be sensitive to its whole field of view all of the time and so would be good at recording dynamic and short lived events.

Hal Anger's first 'gamma-ray camera' of 1952 utilized a scintillating crystal and a pin-hole collimator coupled to a film and he successfully obtained an image of the thyroid but the patients were receiving therapeutic doses of iodine-131. His camera of 1957 became the forerunner of modern nuclear medicine cameras and consisted of a 4×0.25-inch sodium iodide crystal, seven 1.5-inch photomultiplier tubes, and a pin-hole collimator, and with this camera Anger obtained a good quality thyroid scan. The multichannel collimator was described in 1958 which meant that organs larger than the thyroid could be imaged. In 1964

Hal Anger described the 'scintillation camera' with an 11-inch crystal with nineteen 3-inch photomultiplier tubes and an 11-inch diameter and 0.5-inch thick sodium iodide crystal and this considerable increased the clinical utility of the camera. In June of 1958 Anger presented this camera at the fifth annual meeting of the Society of Nuclear Medicine in Los Angeles and for the following 3 years he tried to get manufacturers interested in manufacturing the camera. The first commercial 'Anger Camera' was installed in September 1962 in Ohio State University Hospital.

Part of the success of the Anger or gamma camera can be attributed to the introduction of technetium-99m as a radiopharmaceutical. Radiopharmaceuticals incorporating technetium-99m had been introduced by Paul Harper at the University of Chicago in 1963. Technetium-99m has a half-life of 6 hours and is eluted from a molybdenum generator, and the gamma rays that it emits have an energy of 140keV which is ideal for the Anger camera. The combination of the Anger camera and an ideal radiopharmaceutical was responsible for the rapid growth of nuclear medicine in the 1970s and 1980s. In 1962 W.P. Grove from the Radiochemical Centre in Amersham called the modern radiopharmaceuticals the 'products of the newer alchemy'. The newer shorter-lived isotopes were of considerable advantage over the older radionuclides which had a comparatively long half-life.

The nuclear medicine brain scan was of considerable importance to neuroradiology. In 1972, the year the CT scanner was announced, James W.D. Bull from the National Hospital in Queen Square in London was describing the results that were obtained from the isotope brain scan and stating that its introduction had revolutionized the field of neuroradiology. The isotope brain scan had been introduced in 1963 at the National Hospital and there had been a dramatic increase in the numbers performed with a concomitant reduction in the number of ventriculograms. Edmund Burrows from Southampton was recommending radionuclide brain scanning for acoustic neuroma in 1975 and was obtaining excellent results. Figure 12.7 illustrates a radionuclide brain scan performed on a gamma camera in 1982, 10 years after the CT scanner was announced, and showing a brain tumour.

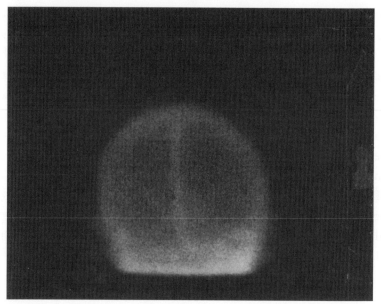

Fig. 12.7 Radionuclide brain scan performed on a gamma camera.
Image courtesy of Dr Adrian M.K. Thomas.

Bone scintigraphy improved in the 1970s and this was significantly helped by the introduction of the new technetium-labelled phosphate compounds, resulting in an increased interest and optimism. In the1970s and continuing into the 1980s the rectilinear scanner was still used for bone scans. In the 1980 it was common for the bone scan to be performed on the rectilinear scanner with gamma camera spot views being obtained of abnormal areas. This was to change with the whole-body gamma camera scan when the single- or dual-headed camera would move on rails along the patient.

Newer agents for imaging were introduced gradually. John Bingham and Michael Maisey from Guy's Hospital described their experience of using DMSA (dimercaptosuccinic acid) in 366 patients in August 1978. This replaced other more invasive methods to determine divided renal function. It is interesting to read early papers of techniques that are now standard techniques in all departments. DMSA was also used to detect pyelonephritic scars in children. By 1980 hepatobiliary iminodiacetic acid (HIDA) scanning was being used in gall-bladder and biliary disease.

Both of these two tests are still in clinical use today. However, it was not obvious at the time which techniques would survive and which would fade away. HIDA and DMSA survive and the use of thallium-201 for the diagnosis of cerebral metastases and selenom-ethionine liver scanning for the diagnosis of hepatoma faded away. There were many developments in the 1980s with the clinical use of indium-labelled white cells in the diagnosis of infection and the intro-duction of the DTPA aerosol system for lung ventilation scanning to diagnose pulmonary embolism. In the 1990s nuclear medicine was in a time of major developments. There were significant developments in radiopharmaceuticals with technetium-99m labelled agents, complex biological agents, and new compounds for labelling with positron emitters. Single-photon emission CT (SPECT) machines continued to improve and positron emission tomography (PET) was becoming more available. In particular there were significant advances in func-tional imaging.

The development of PET and SPECT

SPECT has its origin in the work on David Kuhl and Roy Edwards in 1963 with their Mark I scanner. This system produced a transverse section emission (non-computed) tomogram and used a radionuclide producing a single gamma ray. The scanner used a pair of collimated detectors and by sweeping a spot whose intensity was proportional to the recorded count rate and arranging that the sweep followed to position of the detectors, a simple back-projected tomogram was gen-erated. As technology improved the data could be fed into a compu-ter and reconstructed into transaxial slices in a manner analogous to CT scanning. The Mark IV scanner of 1976 consisted of four detector assemblies that surrounded the brain. The only motion of the scanner was rotational and it was designed to study local cerebral physiology. There were many different types of early SPECT scanners includ-ing the Vanderbilt University Mark 1 and Mark 2, the Harvard Head Scanner, and the Aberdeen Section Scanner. In 1975 John Keyes built the first gamma camera-based SPECT machine, the Humongotron, the first machine to rotate a gamma camera successfully around a patient.

The gamma camera SPECT scanners could be single or dual head and SPECT became standard practice in nuclear medicine departments.

Henry N. Wagner, a pioneer in imaging brain neuroreceptors, has described PET as the most important advance in biomedical science, coming into use just as it was needed to advance the new molecular orientation of biology. This area had been foreseen by William Myers in 1941 who had realized the potential use of positron emitting radiotracers that could be produced by cyclotrons. The existence of the positron (a positively charged electron) had been postulated by Paul Dirac in 1925 and had been shown by Carl Anderson in 1932. When Irène Curie and Frederick Joliot discovered artificial radioactivity in 1934 they were able to identify positron-emitting radionuclides. The first ring system for PET was introduced in 1974 and the first area detector PET in 1968. PET is considerably less available than SPECT because the radionuclides required are produced in a cyclotron. PET scanning has become of increasing usefulness in demonstrating the presence and the location of primary and secondary tumours, depending upon their metabolic rate, and by the late 1980s there were calls for regional cyclotron facilities and lower-cost positron camera systems.

Both SPECT and PET can be combined with CT scanning and systems are available to combine PET and magnetic resonance. CT possesses good spatial localization and the strength of nuclear medicine has always been in its demonstration of physiology rather than anatomy, so by combining the two modalities as a fused image the strengths of both techniques are utilized. Figure 12.8 shows images obtained during sentinel node imaging for breast cancer. The nuclear medicine study identifies the sentinel node and the CT scan anatomically locates the node. These images can now be obtained routinely and SPECT-CT is now the standard for nuclear medicine departments.

Molecular imaging

Techniques continue to develop. Molecular imaging is a development of medical imaging at the intersection between radiological imaging and molecular biology and started in the first decade of the 21st century. Molecular imaging is concerned with visualizing cellular function

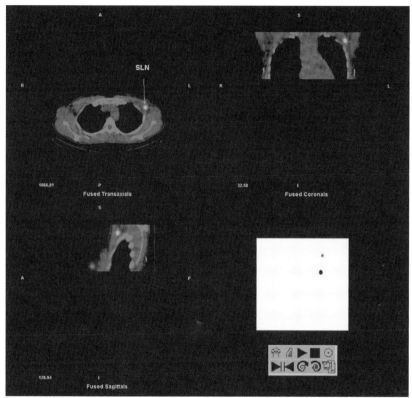

Fig. 12.8 SPECT-CT for sentinel node localization. The nuclear medicine and CT images are fused to facilitate surgical localization of the lymph node. The functional nuclear medicine images are combined with the anatomical CT images.

Reproduced with permission of the South London Healthcare NHS Trust. Image courtesy of Dr Adrian M.K. Thomas.

molecular processes without interfering with them. There are many uses including the investigation of malignancy, neurological disorders, and cardiovascular disease. There is a possible economic impact because of earlier and more accurate diagnosis.

The physicist Max Born told the tale of the typesetter who printed 'unclear science' instead of 'nuclear science'. We have also heard spoken of 'I-suppose-o-topes' instead of isotopes when referring to imprecise nuclear medicine images and reports! However, our modern images are anything but imprecise and are leading to an ever deeper awareness of physiological and pathological processes in disease.

References

1. **Wagner, H.N.** (2006). *A Personal History of Nuclear Medicine*. London: Springer Verlag.
2. **Halnan, K.** (1957). *Atomic Energy in Medicine*. London: Butterworths Scientific Publications.
3. **Brian, D.** (2005). *The Curies: A Biography of the Most Controversial Family in Science*. Hoboken, NJ: Wiley.
4. **Curie, E.** (1938). *Madame Curie*. London: William Heinmann
5. **Curie, E.** (1939). *Madame Curie*. New York, NY: Doubleday.
6. **Rowlands, P. and Attwood, V.** (Eds) (2006). *War and Peace: The Life and Work of Sir Joseph Rotblatt*. Liverpool: The University of Liverpool.
7. **Ansell, G. and Rotblat, J.** (1948). Radioactive iodine and a diagnostic aid for intrathoracic goitre. *British Journal of Radiology*, 21, 552–558.
8. **Mallard, J. and Trott, N.G.** (1979). Some aspects of the history of nuclear medicine in the United Kingdom. *Seminars in Nuclear Medicine*, 9, 203–217.

Chapter 13

Review and the future

The development of radiology has steadily progressed since 1895. In some ways the 1970s can be seen as a golden decade for radiology with the introduction of cross-sectional imaging (computed tomography (CT) and magnetic resonance imaging (MRI)), increased use of ultrasound, and the start of interventional radiology. The advantage of the newer technologies of ultrasound, Doppler studies, and MRI is that they do not expose the patient to the hazard of ionizing radiation. Recording of the radiological image is being moved progressively from the traditional film/screen photographic technique into digital electronic imaging, and thereby permitting extensive manipulation of the data. Many of the traditional radiological procedures using ionizing radiation and contrast media are now obsolete and forgotten.

The role of the radiologist has been gradually changing. In the UK in the early days radiographic reports could be made by anyone and there was no specific qualification required. However, from the 1920s reporting became the provenance of the medically qualified radiologist and radiographers and electrical engineers were excluded. This state of affairs lasted for many years and the professions forgot that anyone other than medical radiologists made reports of radiographic examinations. However, by the 1990s attitudes were changing, and in 1994 Chris Loughran commented on the reporting by radiographers of plain radiographs in cases of trauma, and on the impact of a training programme in clinical reporting. He concluded that such a programme of training and certification of radiographers in fracture reporting could help alleviate the diagnostic radiologist's workload of plain film reporting at a time of increasing pressure on radiology departments. By 1996 it was being recommended that radiographers could be used as second readers in screening mammography. In April 1996 the British Institute of

Radiology (BIR) Diagnostic Methods Committee organized a meeting on skill mix for radiologists and radiographers where this whole subject was discussed and by December 1996 Philip Robinson from Leeds was presenting the results of a feasibility study of plain film reporting by radiographers. In the UK the roles of radiographers has continued to be extended, although in other countries it remains controversial.

The degree of sophistication and insight of the pioneers is quite remarkable. Wilhelm Röntgen, having radiographed his wife Bertha's hand, was soon aware of the wide range of potential uses of his discovery other than for medical indications. These would lead to industrial radiography, non-destructive testing, X-ray crystallography, and X-ray astronomy, as well as to forensic and other uses. In the medical sphere, Charles Thurstan Holland and many others soon realized the very wide range of clinical uses of the discovery. Future developments may increase the sophistication of the examination although we should note that the range of possibilities was already appreciated in the early days of radiology. The trade cards show how complex scientific ideas can be disseminated to the general public and again how later developments develop the early insights and ideas.

The radiological community owes a debt of gratitude to Alban Köhler, Sebastian Gilbert Scott, and Theodore Keats and others who have contributed to our understanding of the normal. Until the normal and its variants are appreciated there will be more false positive diagnoses and inappropriate treatments. With the increasing complexity and sophistication of contemporary medical imaging, the need to understand the normal and its variations becomes ever more important so as to avoid spurious and inaccurate diagnoses leading to unnecessary treatments and conclusions. The possibility for error increases with the complexity of the examinations and this is as true for MRI in 2012 as it was for plain radiography in 1912. In 1159, John of Salisbury wrote in his *Metalogicon* 'Bernard of Chartres used to say that we are like dwarfs on the shoulders of giants, so that we can see more than they, and things at a greater distance, not by virtue of any sharpness of sight on our part, or any physical distinction, but because we are carried high and raised up by their giant size'.[1] We can echo these words and salute the radiological pioneers.

The centrality of medical imaging to modern clinical medicine

The impact of CT scanning on the X-ray equipment industry is interesting. The CT scanner or EMI (Electrical and Musical Industries) scan developed by EMI Medical Inc was quite unexpected by the large X-ray equipment companies and it took them some time to catch up. The X-ray industry had been concentrating on increasingly sensitive X-ray film-intensifying screen combinations with ever finer resolution. The EMI/CT scanner was initially of lower resolution and used an entirely different physical principle. There are stories told of Hounsfield approaching several eminent radiologists with his early ideas and not being greeted with any enthusiasm. It is salutary to consider how the research that led to the CT scanner did not come from the major X-ray companies in the same way that the research that led to our modern low-osmolar non-ionic contrast media did not develop in one of the large contrast-media companies but in a small Norwegian company. In a similar manner, the first paper by Torsten Almén on the idea of a non-ionic contrast agent had no immediate impact in the radiological community and also the significance of the papers of Allan Cormack was not recognized. In the mid-1960s EMI had only a minor involvement in medicine by way of a subsidiary. By the mid-1970s EMI was a world leader in advanced medical technology with a full order book and a significant market potential at that time valued at £100 million per year. The story of the rise and decline of EMI Medical Inc is salutatory and today EMI has no medical connection at all.

In 1978 Louis Kreel edited a book looking at the various leading edges of radiology.[2] There is a perceptive introduction to this book by Robert Steiner who was professor at the Hammersmith Hospital and who had a significant role in the development of cardiovascular imaging in the UK. As Steiner says in his introduction, who would have thought 10 years ago (that is, in 1968) that such momentous developments were possible? Indeed, there were many who believed that diagnostic radiology had reached its zenith and that there was little further room for new innovations. Kreel's book shows how very wrong they were in their predictions. The book came out at the beginning of the applications of these new techniques to clinical practice and it was difficult at the time to predict just how far they were going to advance our ability to establish even more accurate and definitive diagnoses. Robert Steiner from the Hammersmith Hospital predicted that the time would come when medical imaging would produce a reliable *in vivo* tissue diagnosis, possibly on a par with a histological diagnosis of a biopsy. We are not at this stage yet but we are well on the way. He also asked the question: How much further can we go and should we advance our diagnostic refinement even further if these achievements cannot be matched in the therapeutic field? So unless advances in treatment go forward, further diagnostic refinements will be of little help in patient management. He was quite right in saying that there are exciting times ahead for all of us. The words of Robert Steiner bring to mind the words of Thurstan Holland in 1895 when he had thought that surgery had reached the acme of its development.

The 1960s was a time of many changes, both social and scientific. The UK National Health Service had been established for some years and radiology was becoming increasingly complex and expensive. Sir Harry Platt spoke of 'medicine at the crossroads' in 1965 at the middle of the decade and there were strong feelings of uncertainty and frustration in both the medical profession and the country. In some respects we are in a similar position today, and whilst modern medicine has made so many gains it is coming under increasing pressure.

The contributions of the Birmingham radiologist James F. Brailsford (1888–1961) to skeletal radiology were huge and his book on the radiology of bones and joints was highly influential. James Brailsford was active in radiology at an interesting time in its history.[3] The period of the pioneers had passed and radiology was developing as a specialty in its own right. By the 1930s there had developed a systematic interpretation of the shadows cast on the X-ray film. Not only was radiology developing but also there was now specialization within radiology. The early radiologists were involved in both diagnosis and radiotherapy but by the 1930s radiology was dividing into those who primarily specialized in radiotherapy and those who spent their time in diagnosis. It was at this time that James Brailsford's great book on *The Radiology of Bones and Joints* was published. The book was issued in 1934 and Brailsford dedicated it to Sir Robert Jones, the pioneer orthopaedic surgeon who had done so much to develop orthopaedic surgery as a science. In the preface to his book, Brailsford describes how radiography had extended our knowledge of the growth, development, and structure of the bones and joints in both health and disease. Brailsford also realized that the technique of radiography required a specialist both for performing examinations and for image interpretation. It was important therefore that the radiologist took an active part in research, diagnosis, treatment, and determining prognosis. If the radiologist was not involved in these areas then Brailsford foresaw that the radiologist was no more than a qualified technician. Brailsford became deeply involved in defining the professional role and responsibilities of the radiologist.

In the 1970s and continuing ever since, the traditional invasive diagnosis and treatment has been supplanted by modern non-invasive diagnosis and minimally invasive therapy (see Table 13.1).

In the 1980s the technology that had been started in the 1970s was becoming gradually more widely available. However, such technology did not come without a cost. The theme of 'Who needs high technology?' was chosen by Ian Kelsey Fry for his Presidential Address of the BIR of 1983. The 1980s was a time of pressures on resources and the use of expensive medical equipment had to be justified. Ian Kelsey Fry concluded by saying that our patients need high technology and that it is the radiologist's role to ensure that we evaluate the technology properly and that, whenever possible, patients are provided with the level of technology appropriate to their clinical needs. Many traditional techniques passed out of use in the 1980s, being replaced by better and more efficacious modalities. For example, in 1970 42% of antenatal patients had a

Table 13.1 Radiological paradigms

Traditional	Contemporary
Non-invasive and invasive diagnosis, often as an inpatient	Non-invasive outpatient diagnosis
Invasive therapy	Minimally invasive therapy

radiographic examination and this had reduced to 3% by 1980. Also, the oral cholecystogram to diagnose gallstones was replaced by ultrasound and the lumbar radiculogram to diagnose a prolapsed lumbar intervertebral disc was replaced by the CT scanner. However, clinicians do need to be confident about the accuracy of new tests when compared to old and trusted procedures. So in the 1980s when CT of the lumbar spine was being introduced it was common for patients to have both contrast lumber radiculography and spinal CT. As confidence grew radiculography gradually passed out of use. It is interesting to note that when MRI of the lumber spine was introduced there were relatively few patients who had both modalities.

Sadly the major event involving radiation in the 1980s was the accident at the Chernobyl nuclear power station, which took place in the Ukraine on 26 April 1986 at 01.23 local time. For the 1987 Mayneord Lecture of the BIR F.A. Fry reviewed the accident at Chernobyl and the paper still makes chilling reading. The BIR held a one-day seminar as part of its 1987 Annual Congress and the topics included radiation accident management, the establishment of levels for medical intervention, the organization of a specialized centre for medical care, emergency planning for nuclear incidents, and medical preparedness for nuclear emergencies. It is important to put reactor accidents into perspective, however public confidence in all uses of radiation is threatened with every new incident, such as the Fukushima Daiichi nuclear disaster, which took place in Japan in 2011.The topic of increasing public concern about radiation has been reviewed historically by Wade Allison[4] who emphasized that excessive fear of radiation could deny humanity the beneficial effects.

Many of the papers published in the early 1980s still described the use of traditional imaging to investigate patients who today would go straight to cross-sectional imaging (CT and MRI) or to ultrasound. This illustrates that CT scanning was still of limited availability in the 1980s and many hospitals could only acquire a scanner after going to public appeal and do the fund raising themselves. Medical imaging technology continued to advance and these advances have significant effects both on clinical practice and on the economics of medicine.

The issues that were of concern are still with us, such as the effects of delayed reporting of radiographs, which was becoming an issue by the 1980s. As the demands on radiology departments increased in the 1980s there was not a concomitant rise in resources. Progressively radiology department went from being up to date with reporting to having a permanent backlog. Radiology became a victim of its own success, at least in the context of a managed healthcare system.

Another problem resulting from the explosion of radiological techniques in the 1970s and 1980s is the very number of different techniques and resultant uncertainty on the part of clinicians about the best technique for the diagnosis of a particular medical problem. In 1982 Robert Steiner from the Hammersmith Hospital in London reviewed the role of radiology in ischaemic heart disease. At this time Steiner described the integration of many imaging techniques with angiocardiography, coronary angiography, nuclear medicine, CT scanning, and MRI scanning being available. This sheer variety of techniques available for investigating a single disease would be astonishing to a previous generation. To illustrate this point further, the Mackenzie Davidson Memorial Lecture at the BIR for 1985 was given by Torgny Greitz on the topic of diagnostic and therapeutic strategies in neuroradiology. The lecture was profusely illustrated by CT scans (for imaging, treatment planning, and for stereotaxis), 'functional' positron emission tomography scanning, and digital angiography. Of particular interest is the integration of images from different modalities, which was to develop in a major way in the following decades.

In the 1980s the subspeciality of interventional radiology was developing rapidly from its beginnings in the 1970s. By the early 1980s there was a considerable experience of coronary, renal, and peripheral angioplasty. It was also being emphasized that there was a need for close cooperation between the various medical disciplines for both optimal case selection and to deal with any complications. Interventional radiology continued to develop and by the 1990s the endovascular treatment of intracranial aneurysms was common and endovascular repair of abdominal aortic aneurysms was starting to displace surgical intervention. In a similar manner to the development of radiotherapy and radiodiagnosis as separate disciplines, so interventional radiology is separating from diagnostic radiology as a separate discipline. Therefore, in the UK in 2010 interventional radiology was granted its subspecialty status and a new training curriculum was introduced. Following this, in June 2012, there was a joint statement from the Royal College of Radiologists (RCR), the Vascular Society of Great Britain and Ireland (VS), and the British Society of Interventional Radiology (BSIR), acknowledging the significant changes to status and training over recent years. On 16 March 2012, vascular surgery became a specialty, independent of general surgery through an Act of Parliament. The RCR, VS, and BSIR worked together to ensure that each separate organization both supported and endorsed the respective applications.

The new vascular surgery specialty requires a specific curriculum and successful training programmes will offer training to a set of minimum competencies in both open and endovascular surgery. Further development will require close cooperation between vascular surgeons and interventional radiologists. Local applications for training units will be made jointly between departments of vascular surgery and interventional radiology.

In order to assist with this transition, the RCR/VS/BSIR liaison group has been re- established with a remit to scrutinize and update the vascular surgery curriculum and its competencies and consider mechanisms and structures for further training in imaging and interventional techniques.

The BSIR and the VS are committed to working together to provide high-quality care and equality of access to all patients with vascular disease in the UK. The re-establishment of the RCR/VS/BSIR liaison group will underpin this cooperation and help in the development of both vascular surgery and interventional radiology for the benefit of future patients.

In the 1990s CT was increasing being used for the management of the acute patient instead of being seen mainly as a cancer scanner. The trend for the increasing use of CT scanning in the management of the acutely ill patient has continued to accelerate. While the newer imaging techniques produce superb images, their very quality and clinical utility has led to an increasing demand on the service. By the 1990s many were expressing concerns relating to the overuse of radiology. For example, MRI had become one of the most powerful diagnostic techniques for investigating diseases of the brain, spinal cord, and musculoskeletal system and the waiting times were inexorably rising. There were also concerns about the overuse of body CT. The balance between the clinical pressures on our departments and our resources to provide a service will always be in tension. As the 1990s progressed it was being increasing asked 'Is computed tomography of the body overused?' and audit was being recommended. It might be felt that the overuse of medical imaging has no harmful sequels apart from the financial; however, this is not the case. In a recent review Ray Moynihan and others[5] discuss the harm that modern medicine is doing by ever more widely defining the concept of disease and detecting it earlier. They comment that virtually the entire adult population can be classified as having at least one chronic condition. There are shades here of the fantasy surgery of the 1930s described previously when radiologists assisted in the diagnosis of imaginary illnesses such as floating kidneys and visceroptosis (dropped organs). Radiology is now seen as contributing to the problems of overdiagnosis in such conditions as breast cancer, lung cancer, osteoporosis, pulmonary embolism, and thyroid cancer. In the case of pulmonary embolism the increased diagnostic sensitivity of the CT pulmonary angiogram has led to the detection of small emboli that may not require treatment. As the definitions of a disease become ever wider and the threshold for radiological investigations fall, so the potential benefit of any intervention is lower. It is, however, worth bearing in mind that whilst the current and future issues for radiology in resource-rich countries are related to excess, the issues for the less wealthy parts of the world are related to getting access to any medical imaging at all, let alone to complex cross-sectional imaging. These inequalities of health will need to be faced and appropriate actions will need to be taken. Those living in wealthy countries where there is over-investigation and over-medicalization, where scanners now have to be make larger to accommodate the increasing size of patients, need to be aware of the needs of the poorer regions of the planet.

In 1990 BIR President Christopher Hill looked at the future for the radiological sciences and recalled the dictum of Ernest Rutherford that there are only two kinds of science: physics and stamp collecting! Hill believed that the invention of CT came as a considerable embarrassment to most members of the medical physics community since, with hindsight, the principle and possibilities should have been 'obvious' to us all. Now, while reluctant to disagree with Kit Hill, what comes over on reading the work of previous generations is that what is obvious retrospectively is not so obvious prospectively. Hill finishes by saying that the foreseeable future of the radiological sciences will not just be 'more of the same'. An example of this is the development of hybrid operating rooms, which promise to deliver multiple benefits. The hybrid rooms have the ability to shift from a diagnostic or interventional procedure to a surgical procedure and may reduce both procedure and recovery times. The hybrid operating rooms open the way to novel transcatheter therapies and will help hospitals support both subspecialist surgeons and interventional radiologists. This also correlates with the blurring of professional boundaries between vascular surgeons and vascular interventional radiologists. There is a steady growth of these hybrid rooms; however, they are expensive and require careful planning. As an example the hybrid operating room at St. Joseph Hospital Heart and Vascular Center in Orange, California, was especially designed to accommodate cardiac, vascular, interventional radiological, and surgical procedures.

The issues facing the pioneers are strangely similar to our own now. Alfred Ernest Barclay (1876–1949) was one of the greatest British pioneers of radiology, working in both Manchester and Oxford. In 1896 he read in *The Manchester Guardian* about the discovery of X-rays and told his family that a man claims to have discovered a new kind of light that will penetrate solids and show the bones of the hand. Barclay thought this absurd! However in 1912 with fellow Manchester radiologist William Bythell (1872–1950) he wrote the famous book *X-Ray Diagnosis and Treatment*.[6] They commented on the need for doctors to be educated in radiology in order to know when radiology would be of help. They also emphasized the need for radiology to be under medical supervision. Of particular interest is their comment that:

> In writing of the X-rays in diagnosis, other methods are not under considera-tion and are therefore seldom referred to, but we cannot too strongly emphasize the fact that the rays are not, as it were, a new sense added to the other five; they do not in any way relieve us from the necessity of training ourselves in the use of the old-established methods of observation that may be used equally well at the cottage bedside or in the wards. Although by themselves the rays may be of value in diagnosis, yet their range of utility and the accuracy of the information given becomes greater and greater the more we combine the information avail-able from every source. There is no royal road to knowledge, as he will find who attempts to use the X-ray evidence as a short cut to save clinical examination; but if the radiographic method is used as a court of appeal and the results are intelligently correlated with the clinical results, we have not the least hesitation in saying that the value of the X-rays can scarcely be overestimated.[6]

These words have been quoted at length because they remain as true today as they did in 1912, one hundred years ago. Although radiology has become more central to clinical practice since those pioneer days, the principles stated by Bythell and Barclay remain as true today as then. An intelligent combination of clinical findings with the radio-logical results will lead to optimum clinical care, no matter what tech-niques may develop in the future.

References

1. **McGarry, D.D.** (Trans.). (1955). *The Metalogicon of John of Salisbury: A Twelfth-Century Defense of the Verbal and Logical Arts of the Trivium*, p. 167. Berkeley, CA: University of California Press. (Original work by John of Salisbury published 1159.)
2. **Kreel, L.** (Ed.) (1978). *Medical Imaging*. Aylesbury: HM & M Publications.
3. **Kapadia, H., Banerjee, A.K., and Arnott, R.** (2004). The life and work of the Birmingham radiologist Dr James Brailsford 1888–1961. *Journal of Medical Biography*, *12*(3), 128–135.
4. **Allison, W.** (2009). *Radiation and Reason*. York: York Publishing Services.
5. **Moynihan, R., Doust, J., and Henry, D.** (2012). Preventing overdiagnosis: how to stop harming the healthy. *British Medical Journal*, *344*, 19–23.
6. **Bythell, W.J.S. and Barclay, A.E.** (1912). *X-Ray Diagnosis and Treatment: A Handbook for General Practitioners and Students*. London: Henry Frowde, Oxford University Press.

Appendix 1

Early British radiology journals

The British Institute of Radiology and its journals[1]

As little as 4 months following the news that X-rays had been discovered reached London a journal was published, the *Archives of Clinical Skiagraphy*. This has remained continuously in print with the current *British Journal of Radiology* being a direct descendant. Times change, however, and the *British Journal of Radiology* is now a purely electronic journal and published online.

Archives of Clinical Skiagraphy: A Series of Collotype Illustrations with Descriptive Text, Illustrating Applications of the New Photography to Medicine and Surgery, May 1896–1897. This was edited by Sidney Rowland (1872–1917) and was the first radiological journal in the world.

Archives of Roentgen Ray (formerly *Archives of Skiagraphy*). The only journal in which the transactions of the Roentgen Society of London are officially reported, 1897–1915. This journal was the official journal of the Roentgen Society.

Archives of Radiology and Electrotherapy. The official organ of the British Association of Radiology and Physiotherapy, 1918.

Archives of Radiology and Electrotherapy (*Archives of the Roentgen Ray*), 1915–1923.

British Journal of Radiology (BIR Section), *Archives of Radiology and Electrotherapy*, 1924–1927.

British Journal of Radiology (Röntgen Society Section). The journal of the Röntgen Society, 1924–1927.

British Journal of Radiology (New Series) 1928–current. This journal is the amalgamation of the *British Journal of Radiology* (BIR Section) and *British Journal of Radiology* (Röntgen Society Section). It is now published online.

The Journal of the Röntgen Society, 1904–1923. This journal was issued by the Röntgen Society following a dispute with the publisher of the *Archives of Roentgen Ray* and in order for it to have a journal entirely under its control.

The British Electrotherapeutic Society and its journal

Medical Electrology and Radiology. An international monthly review (with which is incorporated *The Journal of Physical Therapeutics*), 1903–1907.

The Royal Society of Medicine and its journals

Proceedings of Royal Society of Medicine (Electrotherapeutic Section), 1907–1931. This journal was the successor to *Medical Electrology and Radiology.*

Proceedings of Royal Society of Medicine (Section of Radiology), 1931–1977.

Journal of the Royal Society of Medicine, 1978–current.

The Royal College of Radiologists and its journals

The Journal of the Faculty of Radiologists, 1949–1959.

Clinical Radiology, 1960–current.

The Royal College of Radiologists currently produces two journals, *Clinical Radiology* reflecting the Faculty of Clinical Radiology, and *Clinical Oncology* reflecting the Faculty of Clinical Oncology.

Reference

1. **Bishop, P.J.** (1973). The evolution of the British Journal of Radiology. *British Journal of Radiology, 46*, 833–836.

Early British radiology societies

The Röntgen Society, founded 18 March 1897. The society was initially named the X-ray Society, and was the first radiological society in the world.[1,2] The society was multidisciplinary.

The British Association for the Advancement of Radiology and Physiotherapy (BARP), founded 1917. The society was responsible for the Cambridge Diploma for radiologists, the Diploma for Medical Radiology and Electrology (DMRE).

The British Institute of Radiology, founded 1924. This society was formed from the BARP.

The British Institute of Radiology incorporated with the Röntgen Society, founded 1927. This society, which continues today, is the amalgamation of the Röntgen Society and the British Institute of Radiology.

The Society of Radiographers, founded 1920. In 1928 the Society of Radiographers was affiliated to The British Institute of Radiology. In 1976 the Society divided into the College of Radiographers to promote professional and educational affairs, and the Society of Radiographers to promote trade union activities.

The British Electrotherapeutic Society, founded 1902. In 1907 this Society joined the 22 medical groups in London in the amalgamation to form the Royal Society of Medicine, and became the Electrotherapeutic Section. In 1932 it become the Radiology Section of the Royal Society of Radiologists.

The British Association of Radiologists, founded 1934.

The Society of Radiotherapists of Great Britain and Ireland, founded 1935.

In 1939 these two groups combined to form the Faculty of Radiologists. At that time it was felt inappropriate to have another medical Royal college and so it was created as a Faculty at, but not of, the Royal College of Surgeons. A charter was granted in 1953, with a further charter in 1975 when the Royal College of Radiologists was formed. In 1990 two college faculties were formed, the Faculty of Clinical Radiology and the Faculty of Clinical Oncology.

The Hospital Physicists' Association, founded 1943. In 1977 the Hospital Physicists' Association was registered as an independent trade union and in 1993 merged with the Manufacturing, Science and Finance Union. In 1982 the Institute of Physical Sciences in Medicine was formed which was concerned with publications and scientific activities, and continues today as the Institute of Physics and Engineering in Medicine.

References

1. **Banerjee, A.K.** (1997). *A History of the Early Years of the British Institute of Radiology: A Centenary Celebration*. London: British Institute of Radiology.
2. **Thomas, A.M.K. and Jordan, M.** (1995). Radiological organisations in the United Kingdom. In Thomas, A.M.K., Isherwood, I., and Wells, P.N.T (Ed), *The Invisible Light. 100 Years of Medical Radiology*, pp. 101–103. Oxford: Blackwell Science.

Appendix 3

Annotated bibliography and reading list

Selected readings in the history of radiology not mentioned in the text:

Anon. (1983). *History of the Hospital Physicists' Association, 1943–1983*. Newcastle upon Tyne: The Hospital Physicists' Association. (An account of the HPA with biographies of the founding members.)

Anon. (1995). *Röntgen Ray Centennial: Exhibition on the Occasion of the Discovery of X-Rays in Würzburg on November 8, 1895*. Germany: Würzburg University. (The illustrated catalogue of the centenary exhibition.)

Calder, J. (2001). *The History of Radiology in Scotland, 1896–2000*. Edinburgh: Dunedin Academic Press.An account of radiology in Scotland.

Carr, J.C. (1995). *A Century of Medical Radiology in Ireland—An Anthology*. Dublin: Anniversary. The development of radiology in Ireland.

Christie, D.A. and Tansey, E.M. (2006). *Development of Physics Applied to Medicine in the UK, 1945–1990*. London: Wellcome Trust Centre for the History of Medicine at UCL. (The transcript of the Wellcome witness seminar.)

Doby, T. and Alker, G. (1997). *Origins and Development of Medical Imaging*. Carbondale, IL: Southern Illinois University Press. (The development of medical radiology.)

Dumit, J. (2004). *Picturing Personhood, Brain Scans and Biomedical Identity*. Princeton, NJ: Princeton University Press. (The development and significance of positron emission tomography scanning on our understanding of the brain.)

Eisenberg, R.L. (1992). *Radiology: An Illustrated History*. St Louis, MO: Mosby Year Book. (A profusely illustrated history covering all aspects of radiology.)

Finch, A. (Ed.) (2012). *Radiating Knowledge: The Story of The Middlesex Hospital Schools of Radiography*. United Kingdom: Disco. (The history of an important school of radiography.)

Geddes, L.A. and Geddes, L.E. (1993). *The Catheter Introducers*. Chicago, IL: Mobium Press. (An illustrated history of interventional radiology.)

Haase, A., Landwehr, G., and Umbach, E. (Eds) (1997). *Röntgen Centennial, X-rays in Natural and Life Sciences*. Singapore: World scientific. (The development of X-rays in science.)

Howell, J.D. (1995). *Technology in the Hospital: Transforming Patient Care in the Early Twentieth Century.* Baltimore, MD: Johns Hopkins University Press. (An account of the impact of technology on the development of the modern hospital.)

Jordan, M. (1995). *The Maturing Years: A History of the Society and College of Radiographers 1970–1995.* London: The Society and College of Radiographers. (The recent history of the Society and College of Radiographers by a former General Secretary.)

Keyles, B.H. (1997). *Naked to the Bone: Medical Imaging in the Twentieth Century.* New Brunswick, NJ: Rutgers University Press. (A history of radiology showing how medical imaging has become a familiar part of modern healthcare and culture.)

Moody, I. (1970). *50 Years of History.* London: The Society of Radiographers. (The early years of the Society of Radiographers.)

Mould, R.F. (1993). *A Century of X-rays and Radioactivity in Medicine, With Emphasis on Photographic Records of the Early Years.* Bristol: Institute of Physics Publishing. (A history of radiology in pictures written by a hospital physicist.)

Newing, A. (1999). *Light, Visible and Invisible.* London: Imperial College Press. (An account of the physical principles underlying the development of radiology.)

Peh, W.C.G. (1996). *101 Years of a New Kind of Rays.* Singapore: Miller Freeman. (Illustrated account of radiology and radiation oncology.)

Del Regato, J.A. (1985). *Radiological Physics.* New York, NY: American Institute of Physics. (A series of illustrated lives of physicists whose work has contributed to medical radiology.)

Roberts, J.E. (1999). *Meandering in Medical Physics: A Personal Account of Hospital Physics.* Bristol: Institute of Physics Publishing. (The life story of a hospital physicist.)

Rodengen, J.L. (2001). *The Ship in the Bottle: The Story of Boston Scientific and the Development of Less Invasive Medicine.* Fort Lauderdale, FL: Write Stuff Enterprises. (The development of a company involved in interventional radiology.)

Rosenbusch, G., Oudkerk, M., and Ammann, E. (Eds) (1994). *Radiology in Medical Diagnostics: Evolution of X-ray Applications 1895–1995.* Oxford: Blackwell Science. (English translation of the German history of radiology.)

Ryan, J., Sutton, K., and Baigent, M. (1996). *Australasian Radiology: A History.* Sydney: McGraw-Hill. (The history of radiology in Australia and New Zealand.)

Tate, A. (1999). *Shadows and Substance: The History of the Royal Australian and New Zealand College of Radiology, 1949–1999.* St Leonards: Allen & Unwin. (The development of the college.)

van Dijck, J. (2005). *The Transparent Body: A Cultural Analysis of Medical Imaging.* Seattle, WA: University of Washington Press. (A study of the cultural and social aspects of medical imaging.)

Van Tiggelen, R. and Pringot, J. (Eds). (1995). *Hundred Years Radiology in Belgium.* Belgium: Belgian Museum of Radiology. (History of radiology from the Belgian Museum of Radiology.)

Index